YOUTH STRENGTH FOR 12-16 YEARS

12-WEEK PROGRAM

ISBN: 9798362640606

Published by www.strengthandconditioningcourse.com

Copyright © 2022 Strength and Conditioning Course Limited

The moral right of this author has been asserted.

All rights reserved. No part of this publication may be reproduced, distributed, or transmitted in any form or by any means, including photocopying, recording, or other electronic or mechanical methods, without the prior written permission of the publisher, except in the case of brief quotations embodied in critical reviews and certain other non-commercial uses permitted by copyright law.

www.strengthandconditioningcourse.com

Facebook & Instagram: **@strengthandconditioningcourse**

Cover Image Copyright: Strength and Conditioning Course

Contents

Contents 2
Introduction 4
Personal Info 5
Goals 6
Strengths and Weaknesses 8
Injury Tracker 8
Key 10
Youth Program Overview 11
Video Tutorials 12
Long-Term Athlete Development 13
    Age 14
    Relative Age 15
    Peak Height Velocity 16
    PHV Tables 17
    PHV Trainability Windows 18
    PHV Considerations 19
    Training Age 20
    Readiness for Max Strength 21
Testing 22
Quantifying Workloads 25
Youth Belt System 26
    Belt Patches 27
    Bodyweight Muscular Endurance Standards 28
    Barbell Strength Standards 29
    Olympic Weightlifting Standards 30
    Speed & Power Standards 31
    Endurance Standards 32
Periodization 33
Strength Program 34
Conditioning Program 35
Strength Warm-Up 36
Conditioning Warm-Up 37
Exercise Selection: Familiarization Phase 38
Exercise Selection: Later Phases 39
Optional/Additional Work 40

How to Use the Log Pages 42
Program Card 1 44
Program Card 2 46
Program Card 3 48
Program Card 4 50
Program Card 5 52
Program Card 6 54
Program Card 7 56
Program Card 8 58
Program Card 9 60
Program Card 10 62
Program Card 11 64
Program Card 12 66
Program Card 13 68
Program Card 14 70
Program Card 15 72
Program Card 16 74
Program Card 17 76
Program Card 18 78
Program Card 19 80
Program Card 20 82
Program Card 21 84
Program Card 22 86
Program Card 23 88
Program Card 24 90
End of Program Tests 92
Final Thoughts 94

Helpful FREE Content! 95

Online Courses 97

Books 99

Introduction

Thanks for purchasing a copy of my Youth Strength and Conditioning Program for 12-16-Year-Olds.

This book works as both a program with detailed instructions and program cards for each training session and a logbook with log pages to track your progress.

Over the next 5-pages, there is room for you to fill in some of your personal information, think about the goals you want to set, consider your current strengths and weaknesses, and log any injuries or ailments you currently have or are affected by.

From there, we get into the program!

First things first:

- Strength Training does NOT stunt growth
- Adolescents can and should be lifting weights
- The stressors of running, jumping, throwing and many sporting actions are often far higher than lifting weights in a controlled manner
- Lifting weights will greatly reduce the risk of injuries during daily and sporting activities
- Lifting weights will benefit an adolescent's physical, mental and social wellbeing and will help to build a more disciplined, motivated and well-rounded individual

Note: An adolescent is generally described as an individual between the ages of 10 and 19.

Personal Info

Name:	
Date of Birth:	
Phone:	
Email:	
Date Started:	

Medical Info:	

Weight, Body Fat Percentage and Girth Measurements (Tape Measure)					
Date:					
Weight:					
Body Fat %:					
Neck:					
Chest:					
Arms:					
Forearms:					
Waist:					
Hips:					
Thighs:					
Calves:					

Goals

There are three types of goals:

- **Outcome Goal(s):** The main goal(s) you are working towards and looking to achieve after a set period of time – the main goal is often referred to as the "overarching goal"

- **Performance Goals:** These are benchmarks you are looking to achieve on your way to the main outcome goal

- **Process Goals:** These are the processes we will take to achieve our outcome goal(s), i.e., I will train 3x a week

Goals are classed as: (these can be adapted to suit you)

- **Short-Term**: 0-1 Month

- **Medium-Term**: 1-6 Months

- **Long-Term:** 6+ Months

Goals should be SMART:

- Specific

- Measurable

- Achievable

- Relevant

- Timed

Short-Term								
Goal:								
Date Set:								
Target Date:								
Achieved:	Y	N	Y	N	Y	N	Y	N

Medium-Term								
Goal:								
Date Set:								
Target Date:								
Achieved:	Y	N	Y	N	Y	N	Y	N

Long-Term								
Goal:								
Date Set:								
Target Date:								
Achieved:	Y	N	Y	N	Y	N	Y	N

Strengths and Weaknesses

Strengths + Notes	Weaknesses + Notes

Injury Tracker

Injury	Notes

Notes

Key

Here are some of the key terms and abbreviations used throughout the program:

- BB = Barbell
- DB = Dumbbell
- KB = Kettlebell
- MB = Medicine Ball
- ES = Each Side
- ED = Each Direction
- OH = Overhead
- SS1 = Strength Session 1
- SS2 = Strength Session 2
- CS1 = Conditioning Session 1
- CS2 = Conditioning Session 2
- RPE = Rating of Perceived Exertion
- RIR = Reps in Reserve
- 1RM = 1 Rep Max – most you can lift for 1 repetition
- 5RM = 5 Rep Max – most you can lift for 5 repetitions
- 1RME = 1 Rep Max Estimation, e.g., Multiply your 5RM by 1.15 (add 15%)
- CM = Countermovement – an initial movement in the opposite direction to which you are jumping or throwing
- CMJ = Countermovement Jump (V = Vertical / H = Horizontal)
- CMT = Countermovement Throw
- Primary Lift = the first strength lift of most importance
- Assistance Lifts = the secondary lifts – help to develop the primary lift or a sporting action
- Concentric phase = muscles shortening – upward phase of a movement
- Eccentric = muscles lengthening – downward phase of a movement
- Steady State = working at a steady pace (low-moderate effort)
- Tempo = working at a continuous set pace – pushing the pace (moderate-high effort)
- Intervals = bouts of high-intensity work followed by rest periods (rest periods are usually longer than the work interval)
- HIIT = High-Intensity Interval Training: Bouts of high-intensity work followed by rest periods (rest periods are usually shorter than the work interval)
- Aerobic = a metabolic process (energy production) that is completed with oxygen: Aerobic Power = how fast energy can be produced / Aerobic Capacity = how long it can be produced for
- Anaerobic = a metabolic process (energy production) that is completed without oxygen: Anaerobic Power = how fast energy can be produced / Anaerobic Capacity = how long it can be produced for
- DOMS = Delayed Onset Muscle Soreness – the muscle soreness felt days after training

Youth Program Overview

This program is designed to develop the Strength and Conditioning of adolescents between the ages of 12 and 16-years-old.

Although there can be disparity between the physical development and maturity of adolescents between the age range of 12-16, this program has been tried and tested across the different age and ability levels and consistently produces brilliant results – the program has been used with complete novices and world-class youth athletes.

The program works through 4x 3-week phases:

1. **Familiarization:** This phase acts as a preload (ease the body into the program), working with moderate volume (how much) and low intensity (how hard). The aim is to develop technique and build familiarity with the fundamental movements.

2. **Accumulation:** This phase increases the volume while keeping intensity low. The aim is to build muscular endurance and an aerobic base (aerobic capacity) – exercise complexity increases.

3. **Intensification:** This phase reduces volume while increasing the intensity. The aim is to build muscular strength, aerobic power and anaerobic power and capacity.

4. **Realization:** This phase reduces volume and increases intensity further. The aim is to build max strength, speed and power.

The initial familiarization phase works on fundamentals and therefore, can be repeated numerous times if necessary.

The program works off 2 Strength Sessions and 2 Conditioning Sessions per week. You can choose to perform all 4 training sessions or any training split that suits you: 2 Strength Only / 2 Conditioning Only / 1 Strength + 1 Conditioning, etc.

Video Tutorials

Video tutorials are available on my YouTube channel: **Coach Jason Curtis**

Here you can find video tutorials for all the fitness tests and strength training exercises, as well as the running, plyometric and ballistic training drills that are recommended.

Web: https://youtube.com/c/coachjasoncurtisacademy

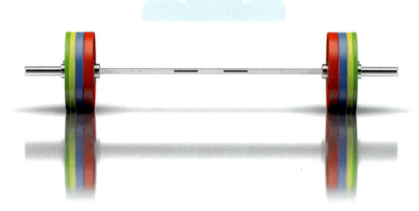

Long-Term Athlete Development

Long-Term Athlete Development, or LTAD for short, is a concept originally designed by Dr. Istvan Balyi.

It is a model or framework for optimal training, competition, and recovery schedules for each stage of athletic development.

There are several LTAD models developed by sporting governing bodies from various nations. However, the 7-stage model below is one of the best examples:

1. **Active Start** – 0-5-Year-Olds
2. **FUNdamentals** – 6-9-Year-Olds
3. **Learning to Train** – 9-12-Year-Olds
4. **Training to Train – 12-16-Year-Olds**
5. **Training to Compete** – 16-18-Year-Olds
6. **Training to Win** – 18+ Year-Olds
7. **Active for Life** – Lifelong Health and Fitness

Within each of these stages, there are **"Trainability Windows"** where the effects of training can be maximized.

It is generally recommended that athletes do not over-specialize early on, but some sports are generally considered to be "Early-Specialization" sports, such as gymnastics, where early specialization can be integral to future success. However, most sports are what can be described as "Late Specialization" sports, such as team sports, where early specialization is not generally seen as a major requirement for future success.

Age

There are several ways we can measure someone's age:

Chronological Age	Biological Age	Somatic Age	Training Age
The clock is set at zero from birth. **Infant:** 0-1 Years. **Early Child:** 1-5 Years. **Mid Child:** 5-8 Years. **Late Child:** 8-Adolescence. **Adolescence:** Puberty **Puberty:** Onset of secondary characteristics **Girls:** 8-19 Years. **Boys:** 10-22 Years	We develop at different stages and rates. **Sexual Age:** The development of secondary sexual characteristics. **Skeletal Age:** This can be measured with a radiograph of the skeleton (wrist).	As biological age is often difficult to measure outside of laboratory settings, somatic methods have been developed using anthropometrics – measurements of body size and proportion. Peak Height Velocity (PHV).	How long has the individual been training and to what level? *Examples:* *Trained for 5 years, once a week at a moderate level.* *Trained for 1 year 6 days a week at a high level of intensity and complexity.* Has the individual got a low or high response to training?

* Individuals can have a high or low fitness baseline (untrained level of fitness), and a high or low response to training (the level of adaptations they experience in response to training). Therefore, no two people will have the exact same response to a training program.

Relative Age

There can be huge differences in two individuals' chronological, biological, and training age. However, there are also other factors to consider.

Biological age measurements can identify an individual's physical development. However, emotional, cognitive, and overall maturity levels also develop at different times and rates (developmental age), and this can impact how ready a young athlete is to partake in competitive settings.

Another huge factor is an individual's relative age, which refers to the difference in age among children who are born in the same calendar year.

The relative age effect (RAE) refers to the phenomenon by which children born early in their year of birth perform more highly than children born later in the same cohort.

In short, some children can be almost a year older (chronologically) than others in the same year. This can create huge developmental differences at a young age and therefore, these children may perform better in a variety of areas. The age gap can result in the older children getting picked for the first team, getting more attention from the head coach, taking part in more training sessions and competing in more competitions, all of which can have a knock-on effect for years to come.

The RAE is one of the reasons why it is key for sports coaches of young children to give all players/athletes a fair amount of attention and game play – only choosing the best players for the team can be detrimental to long-term success (some children require more game time to come into their own but may ultimately become better players – consider an individuals response to training).

Peak Height Velocity

Research has shown that chronological age is not a good indicator on which to base athletic development between the ages of 10 to 16. This is because there is a wide variation in the physical, cognitive, and emotional development within this age group. Therefore, measures such as peak height velocity (PHV) are often used.

PHV is the period of time where the athlete experiences their fastest upward growth in stature (after the 1st year of life, which is the fastest rate of growth).

The average age for reaching PHV is 12 for girls and 14 for boys. Peak weight velocity usually follows shortly after PHV.

Following PHV, VO2 max and strength increase significantly as a result of growth. Most girls experience their first menstrual cycle approximately one year after PHV.

Age of Peak Height velocity (APVH) can be estimated by creating a calculation between: Gender / Date of Birth / Date of Test / Standing Height / Sitting Height / Weight.

Coaches can also start measuring an athlete's height every 3 months from the age of 6. From there, they plot the results on a graph with height on the vertical axis and age on the horizontal axis – see the images on the next page.

Note: The Black blocks show where key Trainability Windows occur – more info on page 18.

PHV Tables

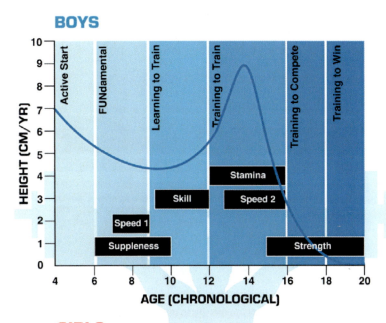

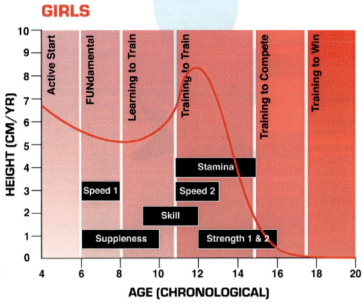

PHV Trainability Windows

Trainability is the responsiveness to training stimuli at different stages of growth and maturation. There are several windows (periods) during a young person's development where trainability is enhanced.

Biological Markers for Developmental Age:

- Onset of PHV (Growth Spurt)
- PHV (After Growth Decelerates)
- Onset of Menarche in Girls

Quality	Trainability
Strength	The optimal training window for girls is immediately after PHV or at the onset of menarche. Whereas for boys, it is 12-18 months after PHV.
Speed	There are two optimal training windows for speed. For girls, the first training window occurs between the ages of 6 & 8 and the second window occurs between the ages of 11 & 13. For boys, the first training window occurs between 7 & 9 and the second training window occurs between 13 & 16.
Stamina	For both genders, the optimal training window for aerobic capacity (endurance) is at the onset of the adolescent growth spurt, prior to reaching PHV. Whereas aerobic power (higher speeds) should be introduced progressively after PHV.
Suppleness	For both genders, the optimal training window for mobility and flexibility is usually between 6 & 10.
Skill	The optimal training window for girls is between 8 & 11. Whereas the optimal training window for boys is between 9 & 12.

Note: Although these are optimal training windows, individuals should be developing these qualities before and after these windows.

PHV Considerations

Although a growth spurt has its pros, such as increased height, strength, and power, it can also have its cons, such as reduced coordination.

During PHV, an adolescent may grow as much as 10cm during the year and therefore, it is clear to see how this could affect coordination.

Injuries can also become more common, both because of reduced coordination and a combination of overuse and rapid growth. The bones are growing faster than the muscles and tendons, which results in the tissues becoming stretched and more prone to strains – some adolescents experience Osgood-Schlatter disease (knee pain) or Sever's disease (heel pain).

It is essential that coaches not only tailor for this by incorporating more ABCs (Agility, Balance, Coordination, Speed), etc. But also that they educate and reassure the athlete that it is a normal part of growth and development – keep the athlete motivated!

Note: If an adolescent experiences persistent pain and discomfort in areas such as their heels, shins, and knees, etc. They should see a medical professional for a full diagnosis – recovery strategies usually involve a reduction in certain activities that are causing negative stress and the implementation of the right strengthening and mobility exercises.

You can download a FREE copy of my 308-Page M&F E-Book

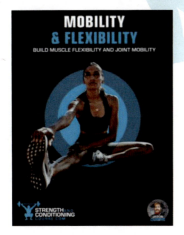

Training Age

Although chronological age can provide basic guidelines and biological/somatic age can provide us with clear indications as to what stage of development the child is in. Ultimately training age can be the biggest factor, especially between adults.

- A 14-year-old who has been strength training 3+ times a week for 4 years is better equipped to handle the stresses of resistance training than a 20-30-year-old who rarely goes to the gym
- A 70-year-old ultra-runner who has been running 26+ mile events for over 40 years is better equipped to handle the stress of ultra-distances than a 20-30-year-old who rarely runs

Training age can be split into two categories:

- **General Training Age:** The number of years spent training and participating in several sports and generalized training
- **Sports-Specific Training Age:** The number of years spent concentrating on 1 sport and practising specialized training

We also consider "**Strength Training Age**" as a specific age, and this is ultimately of most importance when it comes to resistance training.

Note: I usually describe Strength Training Age as the number of weeks/months/years spent following a properly structured strength training protocol/program.

Readiness for Max Strength

Once a young person has learned the fundamentals and has spent 3-8 weeks lifting low-moderate loads, working on technique, and building a solid foundation with higher rep ranges. We can use "**Rep Targets**" to ensure the athlete is not working beyond what their structures can tolerate.

For example, before an athlete attempts to lift 50kg (their perceived 1RM (most they can lift for 1 repetition) they should be able to:

Note: If an individual has no idea of what their 1RM might be, they should spend more time lifting moderate loads to gain experience)

- Perform 10 reps at **70%** of 50kg (35kg) with no breakdown in form
- Perform 8 reps at **75%** of 50kg (37.5kg) with no breakdown in form
- Perform 5 reps at **80%** of 50kg (40kg) with no breakdown in form
- Perform 3 reps at **85-90%** of 50kg (42.5-45kg) with no breakdown in form
- Perform 2 reps at **90-95%** of 50kg (45-47.5kg) with no breakdown in form

The example above is a protocol I came up with to use over 6-weeks: descending the reps each week (10, 8, 5, 3, 2), and then performing a 1RM attempt on week 6.

Note: When working with adolescents, I like them to perform "**Training Maxes**", which involve lifting the most weight with minimal breakdown in form: This number may be 10-15% less than what their true max is, but still provides a good number to program off (often much better than a max that is an absolute grind and executed with huge breakdown in form).

Testing

Before the start of the 1st cycle of the 12-week program, perform 3 muscular endurance tests: Take 3-5 minutes rest between each test.

- **Push-Ups:** 1-Minute Best Effort
- **Sit-Ups:** 1-Minute Best Effort
- **Wall Sit:** Max Time

Note: These exercises are not specifically focused on during the program, but even so, great improvements should be made over the 12-weeks. You can, however, add sit-ups and push-ups in at the end of the workouts (or outside of the gym) – see the optional work on page-40.

Test	Date	Date	Date	Date
	Score	Score	Score	Score
Push-Up				
Sit-Up				
Wall-Sit				

After completing the 1st 12-week cycle, the 3 muscular endurance tests are repeated along with 6 other tests: (instructions on page-92+93)

- **3 Maximal Strength Tests:** Back Squat / Bench Press / Deadlift
- **1 Speed Test:** 100m Sprint
- **1 Endurance Test:** 2km Run or Row

Post-Program Muscular Endurance Tests:

Test	Date	Date	Date	Date
	Score	Score	Score	Score
1m Push-Up				
1m Sit-Up				
Max Wall-Sit				

Post-Program Strength, Speed and Endurance Tests:

Test	Date	Date	Date	Date
	Score	Score	Score	Score
Back Squat				
Bench Press				
Deadlift				
100m Sprint				
2km Run/Row				

Instructions on how to carry out the final testing are on page-92+93

Notes: Other Tests + Scores

An optional test that can be added to the muscular endurance tests at the start and end of the program could be Max Pull-Ups or Chin-Ups if you prefer.

Note: Pull-ups involve having your palms facing away from you, whereas chin-ups involve having your palms facing you – chin-ups are the easier of the 2 exercises.

Quantifying Workloads

This program uses the RPE Scale (Rating of Perceived Exertion) to quantify training loads. This is done by rating the intensity of an activity from 1-10.

The RPE Scale is a subjective measure, meaning it is based on how you feel (not objective data, i.e., a test score). Therefore, it is not a perfect system and does require some experience to understand what equates to an RPE 7 on various activities or exercises, for example, a 2km run or 10 reps of a squat. However, it is by far the simplest way to program and monitor training loads.

Note: You can also give an RPE Score for the entire session – over time, this paints a great picture of how you are feeling throughout the training week.

RPE	Intensity
1-2	Very easy
3	Easy
4	Moderate
5-6	Somewhat hard
7-8	Hard
9	Very Hard
10	Maximal

Another way to evaluate the intensity of a set is Reps in Reserve (RIR), where an individual estimates how many more reps they could perform. For example, and RIR of 2 after a set of 10 squats, suggests they were working at around RPE 9.

Once the first 12-week cycle of the program has been completed and 1RMs are established. Percentages of the 1RM can be used on the primary barbell lifts – I have input my recommended percentage below the programmed RPE score on the program cards.

Youth Belt System

Training shouldn't be boring, so I created a Belt System with male and female standards.

5 Disciplines, 8 Tests Per Discipline (40 in Total), 8 Belts to Achieve!

1. 8x Bodyweight Muscular Endurance
2. 8x Barbell Strength
3. 8x Olympic Weightlifting
4. 8x Speed & Power
5. 8x Endurance

To achieve a belt for a specific discipline, you must achieve all 8 standards.

Gain your True TRIBRID Belt (**Strength** – **Speed** – **Stamina**) by achieving all 8 standards in every discipline (40 tests in total) for a specific colour.

The Youth Belt System is aimed at adolescents between the ages of 10 and 19. Of course, younger children can take part but may find even the White Belt standards out of reach – the Bodyweight Muscular Endurance standards are the most accessible.

The system does not break age categories down because the aim is for participants to progress through the belts as they grow older, faster, fitter, and stronger. There are also no weight categories – greater size may benefit some disciplines but not others.

It is advised that adolescents start with the Bodyweight Muscular Endurance standards. Progress to Speed and Power, work through the shorter Endurance standards and then build up to the Barbell Strength, longer Endurance and Olympic Weightlifting standards.

I have highlighted the Standards specific to this program's tests in **Red**.

Belt Patches

To gain your patches for this program, you need to complete all the program tests (marked in red on the Belt System tables) to the belt colour standard: You can grab yourself a TRIBRID Belt Patch, which are available on my website: www.jasoncurtis.org

For example, if you complete all the programmed tests to the Red Belt Standard, you get a patch with a Red Trim. If you complete all the Blue Belt Standards, you get a patch with a Blue Trim.

If you complete all the Black Belt Standards, you get the TRIBRID Black Belt Patch – if you can achieve that, you are a MACHINE!

If you achieve a TRIBRID Patch (of any colour) tag me in on social media or drop me an email to jay@scc.coach and I'll be sure to give you a shoutout!

Instagram & Facebook: @strengthandconditioningcourse

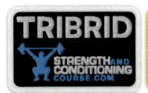 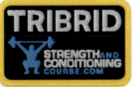 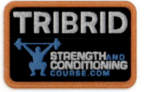

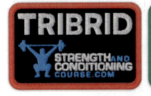 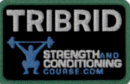 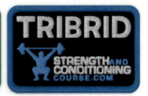

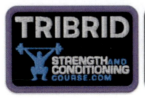 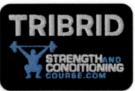

Bodyweight Muscular Endurance Standards

MALE: BODYWEIGHT MUSCULAR ENDURANCE								
TEST	WHITE	YELLOW	ORANGE	RED	GREEN	BLUE	PURPLE	BLACK
MAX WALL SIT	>30s	>1m	>1m 30s	>2m	>2m 30s	>3m	>3m 30s	>4m
1M PUSH UP	10reps	15reps	20reps	25reps	30reps	35reps	40reps	50reps
1M PULL UP	2reps	3reps	5reps	6reps	8reps	10reps	12reps	15reps
MAX DEAD HANG	>30s	>1m	>1m 30s	>2m	>2m 30s	>3m	>3m 30s	>4m
1M SIT UP	15reps	20reps	25reps	30reps	35reps	40reps	45reps	55reps
1M LEG TUCK	6reps	8reps	10reps	12reps	14reps	16reps	18reps	20reps
MAX FRONT PLANK	>30s	>1m	>1m 30s	>2m	>2m 30s	>3m	>3m 30s	>4m
MAX SIDE PLANK	>20s	>40s	>1m	>1m 20s	>1m 40s	>2m	>2m 20s	>2m 40s

FEMALE: BODYWEIGHT MUSCULAR ENDURANCE								
TEST	WHITE	YELLOW	ORANGE	RED	GREEN	BLUE	PURPLE	BLACK
MAX WALL SIT	>30s	>1m	>1m 30s	>2m	>2m 30s	>3m	>3m 30s	>4m
1M PUSH UP	5reps	8reps	12reps	15reps	18reps	21reps	25reps	30reps
1M PULL UP	1rep	2reps	3reps	4reps	5reps	6reps	7reps	8reps
MAX DEAD HANG	>20s	>40s	>1m	>1m 20s	>1m 40s	>2m	>2m 20s	>2m 40s
1M SIT UP	10reps	15reps	20reps	25reps	30reps	35reps	>40reps	50reps
1M LEG TUCK	4reps	5reps	6reps	7reps	8reps	10reps	12reps	14reps
MAX FRONT PLANK	>30s	>1m	>1m 30s	>2m	>2m 30s	>3m	>3m 30s	>4m
MAX SIDE PLANK	>20s	>40s	>1m	>1m 20s	>1m 40s	>2m	>2m 20s	>2m 40s

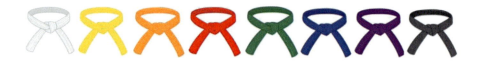

Barbell Strength Standards

MALE: BARBELL STRENGTH								
TEST	WHITE	YELLOW	ORANGE	RED	GREEN	BLUE	PURPLE	BLACK
BACK SQUAT	30kg	40kg	50kg	60kg	75kg	90kg	110kg	130kg
FRONT SQUAT	20kg	25kg	30kg	40kg	50kg	65kg	80kg	95kg
CON DEADLIFT	40kg	50kg	60kg	80kg	100kg	120kg	130kg	150kg
SUMO DEALIFT	40kg	50kg	60kg	80kg	100kg	120kg	130kg	150kg
HEX BAR DEADLIFT	50kg	60kg	70kg	90kg	110kg	130kg	140kg	160kg
BENCH PRESS	20kg	25kg	30kg	40kg	50kg	65kg	80kg	95kg
STRICT PRESS	10kg	15kg	20kg	30kg	35kg	40kg	45kg	50kg
PUSH PRESS	15kg	20kg	30kg	35kg	40kg	45kg	50kg	60kg

FEMALE: BARBELL STRENGTH								
TEST	WHITE	YELLOW	ORANGE	RED	GREEN	BLUE	PURPLE	BLACK
BACK SQUAT	20kg	25kg	30kg	40kg	50kg	65kg	75kg	90kg
FRONT SQUAT	10kg	15kg	20kg	30kg	35kg	40kg	45kg	50kg
CON DEADLIFT	30kg	40kg	45kg	50kg	60kg	75kg	90kg	110kg
SUMO DEALIFT	30kg	40kg	45kg	50kg	60kg	75kg	90kg	110kg
HEX BAR DEADLIFT	40kg	45kg	50kg	60kg	75kg	90kg	110kg	120kg
BENCH PRESS	10kg	15kg	20kg	25kg	30kg	35kg	45kg	50kg
STRICT PRESS	5kg	10kg	15kg	17.5kg	20kg	25kg	30kg	35kg
PUSH PRESS	7.5kg	12.5kg	17.5kg	20kg	25kg	30kg	35kg	40kg

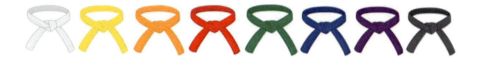

Olympic Weightlifting Standards

TEST	WHITE	YELLOW	ORANGE	RED	GREEN	BLUE	PURPLE	BLACK
MALE: OLYMPIC WEIGHTLIFTING								
OH SQUAT	10kg	15kg	20kg	30kg	40kg	50kg	55kg	60kg
SNATCH BALANCE	7.5kg	12.5kg	15kg	20kg	30kg	40kg	45kg	55kg
SNATCH	5kg	7.5kg	12.5kg	17.5kg	25kg	35kg	40kg	50kg
POWER SNATCH	5kg	7.5kg	12.5kg	17.5kg	20kg	30kg	35kg	45kg
CLEAN	10kg	15kg	20kg	25kg	35kg	45kg	60kg	70kg
POWER CLEAN	10kg	15kg	20kg	25kg	30kg	40kg	50kg	60kg
POWER JERK	10kg	12.5kg	15kg	20kg	30kg	40kg	45kg	55kg
SPLIT JERK	10kg	12.5kg	15kg	20kg	30kg	40kg	45kg	55kg

TEST	WHITE	YELLOW	ORANGE	RED	GREEN	BLUE	PURPLE	BLACK
FEMALE: OLYMPIC WEIGHTLIFTING								
OH SQUAT	5kg	10kg	15kg	20kg	25kg	30kg	35g	40kg
SNATCH BALANCE	5kg	10kg	15kg	20kg	25kg	30kg	35g	40kg
SNATCH	5kg	10kg	15kg	20kg	25kg	30kg	35g	40kg
POWER SNATCH	5kg	7.5kg	10kg	15kg	20kg	25kg	30kg	35kg
CLEAN	10kg	12.5kg	15kg	20kg	30kg	35kg	45g	50kg
POWER CLEAN	7.5kg	10kg	12.5kg	15kg	20kg	30kg	35g	40kg
POWER JERK	5kg	10kg	15kg	20kg	25kg	30kg	35kg	40kg
SPLIT JERK	5kg	10kg	15kg	20kg	25kg	30kg	35kg	40kg

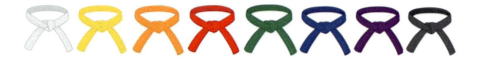

Speed & Power Standards

TEST	MALE: SPEED & POWER							
	WHITE	YELLOW	ORANGE	RED	GREEN	BLUE	PURPLE	BLACK
30M SPRINT	<5s	<4.9s	<4.8s	<4.7s	<4.6s	<4.4s	<4.2s	<4s
50M SPRINT	<9s	<8.6s	<8.4s	<8.2s	<8s	<7.8s	<7.6s	<7.4s
100M SPRINT	<14.5s	<13.5s	<13s	<12.8s	<12.6s	<12.4s	<12.2s	<12s
400M SPRINT	<90s	<85s	<80s	<75s	<70s	<65s	<60s	<55s
VERTICAL CMJ	>20cm	>25cm	>30cm	>35cm	>40cm	>45cm	>50cm	>55cm
BROAD CMJ	>1.7m	>1.8m	>1.9m	>2m	>2.1m	>2.2m	>2.3m	>2.4m
100M ROW	<24s	<23s	<22s	<21s	<20s	<19s	<18.5s	<18s
100M SKI ERG	<24s	<23s	<22s	<21s	<20s	<19s	<18.5s	<18s

TEST	FEMALE: SPEED & POWER							
	WHITE	YELLOW	ORANGE	RED	GREEN	BLUE	PURPLE	BLACK
30M SPRINT	<5.2s	<5.1s	<5s	<4.9s	<4.8s	<4.7s	<4.6s	<4.5s
50M SPRINT	<9.8s	<9.4s	<9.2s	<8s	<8.8s	<8.4s	<8.2s	<8s
100M SPRINT	<15.5s	<14.5s	<14s	<13.8s	<13.6s	<13.4s	<13.2s	<13s
400M SPRINT	<100s	<95s	<90s	<85s	<80s	<75s	<70s	<65s
VERTICAL CMJ	>10cm	>15cm	>20cm	>25cm	>30cm	>35cm	>40cm	>45cm
BROAD CMJ	>1.2m	>1.3m	>1.4m	>1.5m	>1.6m	>1.7m	>1.8m	>1.9m
100M ROW	<28s	<27s	<26s	<25s	<24s	<23s	<22s	<21s
100M SKI ERG	<30s	<29s	<28s	<27s	<26s	<25s	<24s	<23s

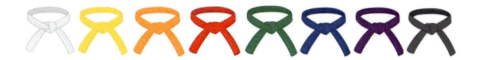

Endurance Standards

	MALE: ENDURANCE							
TEST	WHITE	YELLOW	ORANGE	RED	GREEN	BLUE	PURPLE	BLACK
2KM RUN	<11m	<10m	<9m	<8m 30s	<8m	<7m 30s	<7m	<6m 45s
5KM RUN	<28m	<26m	<24m	<23m	<22m	<21m 30s	<19m 30s	<18m 30s
10KM RUN	<60m	<55m	<50m	<48m	<45m	<42m	<40m	<39m
2KM ROW	<10m	<9m 30s	<8m 30s	<8m	<7m 30s	<7m 15s	<7m	<6m 45s
5KM ROW	<25m	<23m	<22m	<21m	<20m 30s	<20m	<19m 30s	<19m
10KM ROW	<54m	<50m	<48m	<44m	<42m	<41m	<40m	<39m
1KM SKI ERG	<6m 45s	<6m	<5m 30s	<5m	<4m 45s	<4m 30s	<4m 15s	<4m
5KM SKI ERG	<25m	<23m	<22m	<21m	<20m 30s	<20m	<19m 30s	<19m

	FEMALE: ENDURANCE							
TEST	WHITE	YELLOW	ORANGE	RED	GREEN	BLUE	PURPLE	BLACK
2KM RUN	<13m	<12m	<11m	<10m	<9m 30s	<9m	<8m 30s	<8m 15s
5KM RUN	<35m	<32m	<30m	<28m	<26m	<24m	<23m	<22m
10KM RUN	<75m	<70m	<65m	<60m	<55m	<50m	<48m	<46m
2KM ROW	<12m	<11m	<10m 30s	<10m	<9m 30s	<9m	<8m	<7m 30s
5KM ROW	<28m	<27m	<26m	<25m	<24m	<23m	<22m 30s	<22m
10KM ROW	<60m	<55m	<50m	<45m	<44m 30s	<44m	<43m 30s	<43m
1KM SKI ERG	<8m	<7m 30s	<7m	<6m 30s	<6m	<5m 30s	<5m	<4m 45s
5KM SKI ERG	<32m	<30m	<28m	<27m	<26m 30s	<26m	<25m 30s	<25m

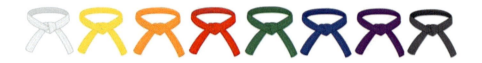

Periodization

The periodization model used in this program uses 4-phases, each consisting of 3-weeks – testing is carried out before and after the program.

The total length of the model is 12-weeks, and this can and should be repeated multiple times to cover the span of a training year.

Phase	Duration	Notes
Testing	Before the Program	1-Min Push-Ups / 1-Min Sit-Ups / Max Wall Sit.
P1 Familiarization	3-Weeks	This phase acts like a preload with moderate levels of volume and low intensity – the aim is to get the muscles working and build familiarity with the movements (develop technique).
P2 Accumulation	3-Weeks	This phase is about building the base with higher volumes and moderate intensity – the aim is to build muscular endurance and an aerobic base (aerobic capacity and power) – exercise complexity increases.
P3 Intensification	3-Weeks	This phase is about upping the intensity and dropping the volume – the aim is to build muscular strength, aerobic power and anaerobic power and capacity.
P4 Realization	3-Weeks	This phase is about peaking for the final test week (or a competition). Intensity increases dramatically (Complex Training), and volume drops significantly – the aim is to build max strength, speed, and power.
Testing	After the Program	Muscular Endurance: 1-Min Push-Ups / 1-Min Sit-Ups / Max Wall Sit. Max Strength: 1RM Back Squat / 1RM Bench Press / 1RM Deadlift. Speed: 100m Sprint. Endurance: 2km Run or Row.

Strength Program

The table below gives an overview of the 12-weeks for the primary and main assistance lifts (some rep ranges may differ on specific exercises, i.e., Lunges).

Phase	Week	Primary Lift (Sets/Reps)	Assistance (Sets/Reps)	Advanced Techniques (Primary Lifts Only)
Familiarization	1	4x6	4x8	N/A
Familiarization	2	4x8	4x10	N/A
Familiarization	3	4x10	4x12	N/A
Accumulation	4	4x12	4x12	N/A
Accumulation	5	4x15	4x10	N/A
Accumulation	6	4x10	4x10	N/A
Intensification	7	4x8	4x8	N/A
Intensification	8	5x5	4x8	N/A
Intensification	9	4x3	4x8	N/A
Realization	10	3x2+2	4x6	Complex Training
Realization	11	4x1+2	3x6	Complex Training
Realization	12	3x1+1	3x6	Complex Training

When it comes to the session plans, all is explained on the program cards. However, if you have any questions about the program at all, drop me an email to: **jay@scc.coach**

Conditioning Program

The table below gives an overview of the 12-weeks for the conditioning sessions.

If performed as a Run, Row of Ski ERG, use the distance as programmed below (meters: rower will be faster than running).

If using a Bike ERG or Spin Bike, double the distances (crank up the resistance on the Spin Bike).

If performing the workouts on an Air Bike using Calories as a metric, perform 10% of the programmed distance.

Phase	Week	CS1 Steady/Tempo	CS2 Intervals
Familiarization	1	1km	4x200m = 800m
Familiarization	2	2km	1x200m + 3x400m = 1400m
Familiarization	3	3km	2x200m + 4x400m = 2000m
Accumulation	4	4km	2x200m + 3x400m + 1x800m = 2400m
Accumulation	5	5km	1x400m + 2x800m + 1x1000m = 3000m
Accumulation	6	6km	1x200m + 2x400m + 2x800m + 1x1000m = 3600m
Intensification	7	5km	1x100m + 2x200m + 3x400m + 1x800m = 2500m
Intensification	8	4km	2x100m + 2x200m + 3x400m = 1800m
Intensification	9	3km	3x100m + 2x200m + 2x400m = 1500m
Realization	10	2km	4x100m + 2x200m = 800m
Realization	11	2km	4x100m + 1x200m = 600m
Realization	12	1km	5x100m = 500m

Strength Warm-Up

The warm-up used within this program is the same for every strength session – doing the same warm-up builds familiarity and once the protocol becomes 2nd nature, it makes for an incredibly efficient warm-up.

Plyometrics (jumps) and ballistic exercises (throws) are performed at the end of the warm-up as potentiation. However, these are specifically programmed at the start of each strength session – optional 2 per session (1 jump, 1 throw).

In this program, we micro-dose (little and often) plyometric and ballistic exercises during the potentiation phase of the warm-up. This protocol raises an individual's arousal levels for the subsequent session and builds reactive strength, power, and tissue resilience over time while reducing the risk of overuse injuries.

Note: Reactive strength is the ability to transition between the eccentric (lengthening) and concentric (shortening) phases of a muscle contraction quickly and forcefully.

Exercise	Sets/Reps/Time	Notes
Run/Row/Ski/Bike	3-6 Mins	RPE 4-5
Bodyweight Squat	1x12	10 Second pause on the last rep (deep squat stretch)
Bodyweight Lunge	1x12	6 Reps with torso rotation and 6 reps with overhead reach
Inchworm to 2x Push-Up	1x5	Crawl out on hands – 2x push-ups – return to standing = 1 rep
Arm Circles & Swings	1x10 of Each	10 Arm circles forward – 10 backward – 10 arm swings

Conditioning Warm-Up

Low-moderate intensity steady state work does not require a specific warm-up (a brief warm-up is still beneficial). However, I highly recommend raising your heart rate and deep muscle temperature prior to any conditioning session where you are pushing the pace – a 200-400m run or row is usually sufficient.

Prior to any high-intensity running session, I highly recommend you perform a pulse raiser and several running drills to reinforce technique and get your structures primed and ready to go – shake off and get a quick breather between each drill.

Below is my standard pre-track session warm-up, which is ideal for any sprint/interval session – of course, you can tailor it to suit you.

Videos for all the below drills can be found on my YouTube Channel:

Coach Jason Curtis

Exercise	Sets/Reps/Time	Notes
Jog	1x200m	RPE 3
High Knees	1x20m	RPE 3-4
Heel Flicks	1x20m	RPE 3-4
Toe Flicks	1x20m	RPE 3-4
High Knee Heel Flicks	1x20m	RPE 5
A-Skips	1x20m	Max Intent
B-Skips	1x20m	Max Intent
Power Skips	1x20m	Max Intent
Bounds	1x20m	Max Intent
Ankle Jumps	1x10	Max Intent

Exercise Selection: Familiarization Phase

The exercises used during the Familiarization phase are introductory exercises that are designed to prepare you for the exercises used during the later phases – the familiarization phase (novice exercises) can be repeated until you can progress to the more advanced phases and exercises (intermediate).

Upon completion of the 12-week program/cycle, you can cycle through it again. On subsequent cycles, you can choose to perform the more intermediate exercises during the Familiarization phase.

Exercises used during Strength Session 1 (SS1): Familiarization

Novice	Intermediate
Goblet Squat	BB Back Squat
DB Lunge (Alternate or Walking)	DB/BB Lunge (Alternate or Walking)
DB Floor Press	BB Bench Press
Standing DB Strict Press	Incline DB Press
DB Lateral Raise	Standing DB/BB Press
Single-leg Calf Raise	Single-leg Calf Raise

Exercises used during Strength Session 2 (SS2): Familiarization

Novice	Intermediate
KB Deadlift	BB Deadlift (Conventional or Sumo)
DB Lateral Lunge	DB/BB Lateral Lunge
DB Bent-Over Row	DB/BB Bent-Over Row
DB Upright Row	DB/BB Upright Row
DB Single-Arm Row	DB Single-Arm Row
DB Biceps Curl + Triceps Extension	DB Biceps Curl + Triceps Extension

Exercise Selection: Later Phases

The exercises used during the Familiarization phase are introductory exercises that are designed to prepare you for the exercises used during the later phases.

Exercises used during Strength Session 1 (SS1): Later Phases

Accumulation / Intensification / Realization
BB Back Squat
DB/BB Lunge (Alternate or Walking)
BB Bench Press
Incline DB Press
Standing DB/BB Press or DB/BB Push Press
Single-leg Calf Raise

Exercises used during Strength Session 2 (SS2): Later Phases

Accumulation / Intensification / Realization
BB Deadlift (Conventional or Sumo)
DB/BB Lateral Lunge
DB/BB Bent-Over Row
DB/BB Upright Row
DB Single-Arm Row
DB/BB Biceps Curl + Triceps Extension

Note: On many of the exercises, you can use dumbbells or a barbell. Use what suits you. However, the barbell is generally the more advanced variation – specialist bars (EZ Bars, Triceps Bars, etc) can be used for exercises like Upright Rows, Biceps Curls and Triceps Extensions, etc.

Optional/Additional Work

For the most part, I want you to stick to the program because the volumes and intensities have been programmed to create progressive overload that will maximize performance, build tissue tolerance and minimize the risk of injury – it is NOT just about how you feel on the day, it is about how that training session will affect the rest of the week.

This being said, time is usually the limiting factor when it comes to including additional work for the core, etc. Therefore, if time and energy allow, you can include the "Optional/additional Work."

Note: **Strength and Conditioning 101 = "What is optimal in the given time and environment"**, which means we want to include the training modes, methods and exercises that pack the most bang for their buck. However, on the flip side, there is a maximum effective dose for any given exercise and therefore, if you do have the time and energy for additional isolation work (single-joint actions), you can add it in.

Here are the core exercises I suggest for the end of any strength or conditioning session: Choose 1-2 exercises – you can also perform 2-3 exercises back-to-back as a Superset (2) or Triset (3).

Exercise	Sets/Reps	Notes
Ab Roll-Out	3x3-10	Increase the intensity by slowing the movement down or pausing at the bottom
GHD Back Extension / Dorsal Raise	3x10-20	Increase the intensity by adding weight or reps
Hanging Knee Raise	3x10-20	Increase the intensity by slowing the movement down
Supine Leg Raise	3x10-20	Increase the intensity by slowing the movement down
Russian Twist	3x10-20 ES	Increase the intensity by slowing the movement down and/or adding weight
Sit-Up	3x10-20	Increase the intensity by slowing the movement down and/or adding weight
DB Woodchop / Band or Cable Rotation	3x10	Increase the intensity by increasing the DB weight or band tension
Pallof Press	3x5-10	Increase the intensity by increasing band tension or slowing the movement down
Front Plank or Push-Ups	3x30-90 Secs	Increase the intensity by engaging your muscles harder
Side Plank	3x30-90 Secs	Increase the intensity by engaging your muscles harder

Jot down any additional exercises you might include		
Exercise	**Sets/Reps**	**Notes**
Pull-Ups	3xMax Reps	Pull-ups are an excellent exercise to add in 2-3 times a week where possible: They can be regressed by using a resistance band or progressed by adding wight with a dip belt – if using a resistance band, stick to a band tension that allows you to do 3-5 reps (keep the intensity high)

How to Use the Log Pages

Note: The Program Log pages have been left blank to allow for exercise variations, etc. There is also space to include warm-up/extra sets – the same exercise can continue onto the 2nd row to allow up to 10 sets.

Step 1: Input the date, day, and time.

Step 2: Input your readiness scores – "Good" soreness = no soreness.

Step 3: Input the exercise names.

Step 4: Warm-up appropriately for the training session.

Step 5: Work up to a weight that feels about right for the programmed intensity.

Step 6: Input the weight you lifted in the top box.

Step 7: Input the reps performed (this is programmed on the program card, but you may perform a different number).

Step 8: Input the RPE score for the set – how hard you felt it was out of 10.

Step 9: Input any miscellaneous notes or notes on metabolic conditioning if performed within the strength session.

Step 10: Input the session RPE (score for the whole session).

Note: If conditioning is performed, input notes in the "Conditioning / Notes" section. If performed on a different day to the strength session, input the date of the conditioning session in the box to start – readiness scores for both strength and conditioning sessions can be completed separately (see example).

See an example on the following page.

Program Log Example: Date: ____ / ____ / ____ Day: _____ Time: _____

Exercise	Set 1		Set 2		Set 3		Set 4		Set 5	
	WEIGHT		*WEIGHT*		*WEIGHT*		*WEIGHT*		*WEIGHT*	
	REP	*RPE*	*REP*	*RPE*	*REP*	*RPE*	*REP*	*RPE*	*REP*	*RPE*
EXAMPLE	120		120							
	10	7	10	8						

Conditioning / Notes	Readiness	Bad	Ok	Good
Input the date of the conditioning session if different to the strength session and fill out the readiness scores for each training session separately: Denote an "S" for Strength and a "C" for Conditioning – see the soreness box for an example.	Sleep:		✓	
	Energy:			✓
	Mood:			✓
	Soreness:	S	C	

Session RPE: _____

Program Card 1

Phase 1: Familiarization – Week-1

Strength Session 1 (SS1):

Aim to be on your working sets on the primary lift within 3-4 warm-up sets. On Assistance lifts, you can perform 1-2 warm-up sets to groove the movements (if needed).

Exercise	Sets/Reps	Intensity	Rest	Notes
Optional: Vertical CM Jump	4x1	Max Intent	5-10 Secs	Jump as high as you can
Optional: MB CM Chest Throw	4x1	Max Intent	5-10 Secs	Use a 3-5kg MB
Goblet Squat	4x6	RPE 5	1-2 Mins	Work on technique
DB Lunge	4x4 ES	RPE 5	1-2 Mins	Alternate or walking
DB Floor Press	4x6	RPE 5	1-2 Mins	Work on technique
Standing DB Strict Press	4x8	RPE 5	1-2 Mins	Work on technique
DB Lateral Raise	4x8	RPE 5	1-2 Mins	Work on technique
Single-Leg Calf Raise	3xMax ES	RPE 10	5-10 Secs	Perform with a heel drop
		RPE 5	10-30 Secs	Optional Core: Your choice from page-40

Conditioning Session 1 (CS1):

Activity	Description: Steady State
Run, Row, etc	1km – RPE 3

Program Log 1: Date: ____ / ____ / ____ Day: _____ Time: _____

Exercise	Set 1 WEIGHT		Set 2 WEIGHT		Set 3 WEIGHT		Set 4 WEIGHT		Set 5 WEIGHT	
	REP	*RPE*	*REP*	*RPE*	*REP*	*RPE*	*REP*	*RPE*	*REP*	*RPE*

Conditioning / Notes	Readiness	Bad	Ok	Good
	Sleep:			
	Energy:			
	Mood:			
	Soreness:			

Session RPE: _____

45

Program Card 2

Phase 1: Familiarization – Week-1

Strength Session 2 (SS2):

Aim to be on your working sets on the primary lift within 3-4 warm-up sets. On Assistance lifts, you can perform 1-2 warm-up sets to groove the movements (if needed).

Exercise	Sets/Reps	Intensity	Rest	Notes
Optional: Horizontal CM Jump	4x1	Max Intent	5-10 Secs	Jump as far as you can
Optional: MB CM Rotational Throw	3x1 ES	Max Intent	5-10 Secs	Use a 3-5kg MB
KB Deadlift	4x6	RPE 5	1-2 Mins	Work on technique
DB Lateral Lunge	4x4 ES	RPE 5	1-2 Mins	Alternate
DB Bent-Over Row	4x8	RPE 5	1-2 Mins	Work on technique
DB Upright Row	4x8	RPE 5	1-2 Mins	Work on technique
DB Single-Arm Row	4x8	RPE 5	1-2 Mins	Work on technique
DB Biceps Curl + Triceps Extension	4x8+8	RPE 5	1-2 Mins	Take 5-10 seconds rest between the two exercises – 1-2 deep breaths
		RPE 5	10-30 Secs	Optional Core: Your choice from page-40

Conditioning Session 2 (CS2):

Activity	Description: Intervals	Rest
Run, Row, etc	4x200m – RPE 6	2-3 Mins
Total Distance	800m	N/A

Program Log 2: Date: ___ / ___ / ___ Day: _____ Time: _____

Exercise	Set 1 WEIGHT		Set 2 WEIGHT		Set 3 WEIGHT		Set 4 WEIGHT		Set 5 WEIGHT	
	REP	RPE	REP	RPE	REP	RPE	REP	RPE	REP	RPE

Conditioning / Notes	Readiness	Bad	Ok	Good
	Sleep:			
	Energy:			
	Mood:			
	Soreness:			

Session RPE: _____

Program Card 3

Phase 1: Familiarization – Week-2

Strength Session 1 (SS1):

Aim to be on your working sets on the primary lift within 3-4 warm-up sets. On Assistance lifts, you can perform 1-2 warm-up sets to groove the movements (if needed).

Exercise	Sets/Reps	Intensity	Rest	Notes
Optional: Vertical CM Jump	4x1	Max Intent	5-10 Secs	Jump as high as you can
Optional: MB CM Chest Throw	4x1	Max Intent	5-10 Secs	Use a 3-5kg MB
Goblet Squat	4x8	RPE 5	1-2 Mins	Work on technique
DB Lunge	4x6 ES	RPE 5	1-2 Mins	Alternate or walking
DB Floor Press	4x8	RPE 5	1-2 Mins	Work on technique
Standing DB Strict Press	4x10	RPE 5	1-2 Mins	Work on technique
DB Lateral Raise	4x10	RPE 5	1-2 Mins	Work on technique
Single-Leg Calf Raise	3xMax ES	RPE 10	5-10 Secs	Perform with a heel drop
		RPE 5	10-30 Secs	Optional Core: Your choice from page-40

Conditioning Session 1 (CS1):

Activity	Description: Steady State
Run, Row, etc	2km – RPE 3-4

Program Log 3: Date: ___ / ___ / ___ Day: _____ Time: _____

Exercise	Set 1		Set 2		Set 3		Set 4		Set 5	
	WEIGHT		*WEIGHT*		*WEIGHT*		*WEIGHT*		*WEIGHT*	
	REP	*RPE*	*REP*	*RPE*	*REP*	*RPE*	*REP*	*RPE*	*REP*	*RPE*

Conditioning / Notes	Readiness	Bad	Ok	Good
	Sleep:			
	Energy:			
	Mood:			
	Soreness:			

Session RPE: _____

Program Card 4

Phase 1: Familiarization – Week-2

Strength Session 2 (SS2):

Aim to be on your working sets on the primary lift within 3-4 warm-up sets. On Assistance lifts, you can perform 1-2 warm-up sets to groove the movements (if needed).

Exercise	Sets/Reps	Intensity	Rest	Notes
Optional: Horizontal CM Jump	4x1	Max Intent	5-10 Secs	Jump as far as you can
Optional: MB CM Rotational Throw	3x1 ES	Max Intent	5-10 Secs	Use a 3-5kg MB
KB Deadlift	4x8	RPE 5	1-2 Mins	Work on technique
DB Lateral Lunge	4x5 ES	RPE 5	1-2 Mins	Alternate
DB Bent-Over Row	4x10	RPE 5	1-2 Mins	Work on technique
DB Upright Row	4x10	RPE 5	1-2 Mins	Work on technique
DB Single-Arm Row	4x10	RPE 5	1-2 Mins	Work on technique
DB Biceps Curl + Triceps Extension	4x10+10	RPE 5	1-2 Mins	Take 5-10 seconds rest between the two exercises – 1-2 deep breaths
		RPE 5	10-30 Secs	Optional Core: Your choice from page-40

Conditioning Session 2 (CS2):

Activity	Description: Intervals	Rest
Run, Row, etc	1x200m – RPE 6	2-3 Mins
	3x400 – RPE 4	3 Mins
Total Distance	1400m	N/A

Program Log 4: Date: ____ / ____ / ____ Day: _____ Time: _____

Exercise	Set 1		Set 2		Set 3		Set 4		Set 5	
	WEIGHT		*WEIGHT*		*WEIGHT*		*WEIGHT*		*WEIGHT*	
	REP	RPE	REP	RPE	REP	RPE	REP	RPE	REP	RPE

Conditioning / Notes	Readiness	Bad	Ok	Good
	Sleep:			
	Energy:			
	Mood:			
	Soreness:			

Session RPE: _____

Program Card 5

Phase 1: Familiarization – Week-3

Strength Session 1 (SS1):

Aim to be on your working sets on the primary lift within 3-4 warm-up sets. On Assistance lifts, you can perform 1-2 warm-up sets to groove the movements (if needed).

Exercise	Sets/Reps	Intensity	Rest	Notes
Optional: Vertical CM Jump	4x1	Max Intent	5-10 Secs	Jump as high as you can
Optional: MB CM Chest Throw	4x1	Max Intent	5-10 Secs	Use a 3-5kg MB
Goblet Squat	4x10	RPE 5-6	1-2 Mins	Work on technique
DB Lunge	4x8 ES	RPE 5-6	1-2 Mins	Alternate or walking
DB Floor Press	4x10	RPE 5-6	1-2 Mins	Work on technique
Standing DB Strict Press	4x12	RPE 5-6	1-2 Mins	Work on technique
DB Lateral Raise	4x12	RPE 5-6	1-2 Mins	Work on technique
Single-Leg Calf Raise	3xMax ES	RPE 10	5-10 Secs	Perform with a heel drop
		RPE 5	10-30 Secs	Optional Core: Your choice from page-40

Conditioning Session 1 (CS1):

Activity	Description: Steady State
Run, Row, etc	3km – RPE 4

Program Log 5: Date: ____ / ____ / ____ Day: _____ Time: _____

Exercise	Set 1			Set 2			Set 3			Set 4			Set 5		
	WEIGHT			*WEIGHT*			*WEIGHT*			*WEIGHT*			*WEIGHT*		
	REP	*RPE*		*REP*	*RPE*		*REP*	*RPE*		*REP*	*RPE*		*REP*	*RPE*	

Conditioning / Notes	Readiness	Bad	Ok	Good
	Sleep:			
	Energy:			
	Mood:			
	Soreness:			

Session RPE: _____

Program Card 6

Phase 1: Familiarization – Week-3

Strength Session 2 (SS2):

Aim to be on your working sets on the primary lift within 3-4 warm-up sets. On Assistance lifts, you can perform 1-2 warm-up sets to groove the movements (if needed).

Exercise	Sets/Reps	Intensity	Rest	Notes
Optional: Horizontal CM Jump	4x1	Max Intent	5-10 Secs	Jump as far as you can
Optional: MB CM Rotational Throw	3x1 ES	Max Intent	5-10 Secs	Use a 3-5kg MB
KB Deadlift	4x10	RPE 5-6	1-2 Mins	Work on technique
DB Lateral Lunge	4x6 ES	RPE 5-6	1-2 Mins	Alternate
DB Bent-Over Row	4x12	RPE 5-6	1-2 Mins	Work on technique
DB Upright Row	4x12	RPE 5-6	1-2 Mins	Work on technique
DB Single-Arm Row	4x12	RPE 5-6	1-2 Mins	Work on technique
DB Biceps Curl + Triceps Extension	4x12+12	RPE 5-6	1-2 Mins	Take 5-10 seconds rest between the two exercises – 1-2 deep breaths
		RPE 5	10-30 Secs	Optional Core: Your choice from page-40

Conditioning Session 2 (CS2):

Activity	Description: Intervals	Rest
Run, Row, etc	2x200m – RPE 6	2-3 Mins
	4x400 – RPE 5	3 Mins
Total Distance	2000m	N/A

Program Log 6: Date: ____ / ____ / ____ Day: _____ Time: _____

Exercise	Set 1 WEIGHT		Set 2 WEIGHT		Set 3 WEIGHT		Set 4 WEIGHT		Set 5 WEIGHT	
	REP	RPE	REP	RPE	REP	RPE	REP	RPE	REP	RPE

Conditioning / Notes	Readiness	Bad	Ok	Good
	Sleep:			
	Energy:			
	Mood:			
	Soreness:			

Session RPE: _____

Program Card 7

Phase 2: Accumulation – Week-1 (week-4 of the program)

Strength Session 1 (SS1):

Aim to be on your working sets on the primary lift within 3-4 warm-up sets. On Assistance lifts, you can perform 1-2 warm-up sets to groove the movements (if needed).

Exercise	Sets/Reps	Intensity	Rest	Notes
Optional: Vertical CM Jump	4x2	Max Intent	5-10 Secs	Jump as high as you can – 2 jumps in quick succession
Optional: MB CM Chest Throw	4x1	Max Intent	5-10 Secs	Use a 3-5kg MB
BB Back Squat	4x12	RPE 5-6 50-55%	1-2 Mins	Work on technique
DB/BB Lunge	4x10 ES	RPE 5-6	1-2 Mins	Alternate or walking
BB Bench Press	4x12	RPE 5-6 50-55%	1-2 Mins	Work on technique
Incline DB Press	4x12	RPE 5-6	1-2 Mins	Work on technique
Standing DB/BB Press	4x12	RPE 5-6	1-2 Mins	Work on technique
Single-Leg Calf Raise	3xMax ES	RPE 10	5-10 Secs	Perform with a heel drop
		RPE 5	10-30 Secs	Optional Core: Your choice from page-40

Conditioning Session 1 (CS1):

Activity	Description: Steady State
Run, Row, etc	4km – RPE 5

Program Log 7:   Date: ____ / ____ / ____   Day: _____   Time: _____

Exercise	Set 1 WEIGHT		Set 2 WEIGHT		Set 3 WEIGHT		Set 4 WEIGHT		Set 5 WEIGHT	
	REP	RPE	REP	RPE	REP	RPE	REP	RPE	REP	RPE

Conditioning / Notes	Readiness	Bad	Ok	Good
	Sleep:			
	Energy:			
	Mood:			
	Soreness:			

Session RPE: _____

Program Card 8

Phase 2: Accumulation – Week-1 (week-4 of the program)

Strength Session 2 (SS2):

Aim to be on your working sets on the primary lift within 3-4 warm-up sets. On Assistance lifts, you can perform 1-2 warm-up sets to groove the movements (if needed).

Exercise	Sets/Reps	Intensity	Rest	Notes
Optional: Horizontal CM Jump	4x2	Max Intent	5-10 Secs	Jump as far as you can – 2 jumps in quick succession
Optional: MB CM Rotational Throw	3x1 ES	Max Intent	5-10 Secs	Use a 3-5kg MB
BB Deadlift	4x12	RPE 5-6 50-55%	1-2 Mins	Work on technique
DB/BB Lateral Lunge	4x6 ES	RPE 5-6	1-2 Mins	Alternate
DB/BB Bent-Over Row	4x12	RPE 5-6	1-2 Mins	Work on technique
DB/BB Upright Row	4x12	RPE 5-6	1-2 Mins	Work on technique
DB Single-Arm Row	4x12	RPE 5-6	1-2 Mins	Work on technique
DB/BB Biceps Curl + Triceps Extension	4x12+12	RPE 5-6	1-2 Mins	Take 5-10 seconds rest between the two exercises – 1-2 deep breaths
		RPE 5	10-30 Secs	Optional Core: Your choice from page-40

Conditioning Session 2 (CS2):

Activity	Description: Intervals	Rest
Run, Row, etc	2x200m – RPE 6	2-3 Mins
	3x400 – RPE 5	3 Mins
	1x800m – RPE 4	N/A
Total Distance	2400m	N/A

Program Log 8: Date: ____ / ____ / ____ Day: _____ Time: _____

Exercise	Set 1		Set 2		Set 3		Set 4		Set 5	
	WEIGHT		*WEIGHT*		*WEIGHT*		*WEIGHT*		*WEIGHT*	
	REP	*RPE*	*REP*	*RPE*	*REP*	*RPE*	*REP*	*RPE*	*REP*	*RPE*

Conditioning / Notes	Readiness	Bad	Ok	Good
	Sleep:			
	Energy:			
	Mood:			
	Soreness:			

Session RPE: _____

Program Card 9

Phase 2: Accumulation – Week-2 (week-5 of the program)

Strength Session 1 (SS1):

Aim to be on your working sets on the primary lift within 3-4 warm-up sets. On Assistance lifts, you can perform 1-2 warm-up sets to groove the movements (if needed).

Exercise	Sets/Reps	Intensity	Rest	Notes
Optional: Vertical CM Jump	4x2	Max Intent	5-10 Secs	Jump as high as you can – 2 jumps in quick succession
Optional: MB CM Chest Throw	4x1	Max Intent	5-10 Secs	Use a 3-5kg MB
BB Back Squat	4x15	RPE 6-7 50-55%	2-3 Mins	Work on technique
DB/BB Lunge	4x10 ES	RPE 6-7	1-2 Mins	Alternate or walking
BB Bench Press	4x15	RPE 6-7 50-55%	2-3 Mins	Work on technique
Incline DB Press	4x10	RPE 6-7	1-2 Mins	Work on technique
Standing DB/BB Press	4x10	RPE 6-7	1-2 Mins	Work on technique
Single-Leg Calf Raise	3xMax ES	RPE 10	5-10 Secs	Perform with a heel drop
		RPE 6	10-30 Secs	Optional Core: Your choice from page-40

Conditioning Session 1 (CS1):

Activity	Description: Steady State
Run, Row, etc	5km – RPE 6

Program Log 9: Date: ____ / ____ / ____ Day: _____ Time: _____

Exercise	Set 1 WEIGHT		Set 2 WEIGHT		Set 3 WEIGHT		Set 4 WEIGHT		Set 5 WEIGHT	
	REP	RPE	REP	RPE	REP	RPE	REP	RPE	REP	RPE

Conditioning / Notes	Readiness	Bad	Ok	Good
	Sleep:			
	Energy:			
	Mood:			
	Soreness:			

Session RPE: _____

Program Card 10

Phase 2: Accumulation – Week-2 (week-5 of the program)

Strength Session 2 (SS2):

Aim to be on your working sets on the primary lift within 3-4 warm-up sets. On Assistance lifts, you can perform 1-2 warm-up sets to groove the movements (if needed).

Exercise	Sets/Reps	Intensity	Rest	Notes
Optional: Horizontal CM Jump	4x2	Max Intent	5-10 Secs	Jump as far as you can – 2 jumps in quick succession
Optional: MB CM Rotational Throw	3x1 ES	Max Intent	5-10 Secs	Use a 3-5kg MB
BB Deadlift	4x15	RPE 6-7 50-55%	2-3 Mins	Work on technique
DB/BB Lateral Lunge	4x5 ES	RPE 6-7	1-2 Mins	Alternate
DB/BB Bent-Over Row	4x10	RPE 6-7	1-2 Mins	Work on technique
DB/BB Upright Row	4x10	RPE 6-7	1-2 Mins	Work on technique
DB Single-Arm Row	4x10	RPE 6-7	1-2 Mins	Work on technique
DB/BB Biceps Curl + Triceps Extension	4x10+10	RPE 6-7	1-2 Mins	Take 5-10 seconds rest between the two exercises – 1-2 deep breaths
		RPE 6	10-30 Secs	Optional Core: Your choice from page-40

Conditioning Session 2 (CS2):

Activity	Description: Intervals	Rest
Run, Row, etc	1x400m – RPE 7	2-3 Mins
	2x800 – RPE 6	3 Mins
	1x1000m – RPE 6	N/A
Total Distance	3000m	N/A

Program Log 10: Date: ____ / ____ / ____ Day: _____ Time: _____

Exercise	Set 1 WEIGHT		Set 2 WEIGHT		Set 3 WEIGHT		Set 4 WEIGHT		Set 5 WEIGHT	
	REP	RPE	REP	RPE	REP	RPE	REP	RPE	REP	RPE

Conditioning / Notes	Readiness	Bad	Ok	Good
	Sleep:			
	Energy:			
	Mood:			
	Soreness:			

Session RPE: _____

Program Card 11

Phase 2: Accumulation – Week-3 (week-6 of the program)

Strength Session 1 (SS1):

Aim to be on your working sets on the primary lift within 3-4 warm-up sets. On Assistance lifts, you can perform 1-2 warm-up sets to groove the movements (if needed).

Exercise	Sets/Reps	Intensity	Rest	Notes
Optional: Vertical CM Jump	3x3	Max Intent	5-10 Secs	Jump as high as you can – 3 jumps in quick succession
Optional: MB CM Chest Throw	4x1	Max Intent	5-10 Secs	Use a 3-5kg MB
BB Back Squat	4x10	RPE 7 60-65%	2-3 Mins	Work at a steady tempo (lift speed)
DB/BB Lunge	4x10 ES	RPE 7	1-2 Mins	Work at a steady tempo (lift speed)
BB Bench Press	4x10	RPE 7 60-65%	2-3 Mins	Work at a steady tempo (lift speed)
Incline DB Press	4x10	RPE 7	1-2 Mins	Work at a steady tempo (lift speed)
Standing DB/BB Press	4x10	RPE 7	1-2 Mins	Work at a steady tempo (lift speed)
Single-Leg Calf Raise	3xMax ES	RPE 10	5-10 Secs	Perform with a heel drop
		RPE 5	10-30 Secs	Optional Core: Your choice from page-40

Conditioning Session 1 (CS1):

Activity	Description: Steady State
Run, Row, etc	6km – RPE 6-7

Program Log 11: Date: ____ / ____ / ____ Day: _____ Time: _____

Exercise	Set 1 WEIGHT		Set 2 WEIGHT		Set 3 WEIGHT		Set 4 WEIGHT		Set 5 WEIGHT	
	REP	RPE	REP	RPE	REP	RPE	REP	RPE	REP	RPE

Conditioning / Notes	Readiness	Bad	Ok	Good
	Sleep:			
	Energy:			
	Mood:			
	Soreness:			

Session RPE: _____

Program Card 12

Phase 2: Accumulation – Week-3 (week-6 of the program)

Strength Session 2 (SS2):

Aim to be on your working sets on the primary lift within 3-4 warm-up sets. On Assistance lifts, you can perform 1-2 warm-up sets to groove the movements (if needed).

Exercise	Sets/Reps	Intensity	Rest	Notes
Optional: Horizontal CM Jump	3x3	Max Intent	5-10 Secs	Jump as far as you can – 3 jumps in quick succession
Optional: MB CM Rotational Throw	3x1 ES	Max Intent	5-10 Secs	Use a 3-5kg MB
BB Deadlift	4x10	RPE 7 60-65%	2-3 Mins	Work at a steady tempo (lift speed)
DB/BB Lateral Lunge	4x5 ES	RPE 7	1-2 Mins	Work at a steady tempo (lift speed)
DB/BB Bent-Over Row	4x10	RPE 7	1-2 Mins	Work at a steady tempo (lift speed)
DB/BB Upright Row	4x10	RPE 7	1-2 Mins	Work at a steady tempo (lift speed)
DB Single-Arm Row	4x10	RPE 7	1-2 Mins	Work at a steady tempo (lift speed)
DB/BB Biceps Curl + Triceps Extension	4x10+10	RPE 7	1-2 Mins	Take 5-10 seconds rest between the two exercises – 1-2 deep breaths
		RPE 6	10-30 Secs	Optional Core: Your choice from page-40

Conditioning Session 2 (CS2):

Activity	Description: Intervals	Rest
Run, Row, etc	1x200m – RPE 7	2-3 Mins
	2x400 – RPE 6	3 Mins
	2x800m – RPE 6	3 Min
	1x1000m	N/A
Total Distance	3600m	N/A

Program Log 12: Date: ____ / ____ / ____ Day: _____ Time: _____

Exercise	Set 1 WEIGHT		Set 2 WEIGHT		Set 3 WEIGHT		Set 4 WEIGHT		Set 5 WEIGHT	
	REP	RPE	REP	RPE	REP	RPE	REP	RPE	REP	RPE

Conditioning / Notes	Readiness	Bad	Ok	Good
	Sleep:			
	Energy:			
	Mood:			
	Soreness:			

Session RPE: _____

Program Card 13

Phase 3: Intensification – Week-1 (week-7 of the program)

Strength Session 1 (SS1):

Aim to be on your working sets on the primary lift within 3-4 warm-up sets. On Assistance lifts, you can perform 1-2 warm-up sets to groove the movements (if needed).

Exercise	Sets/Reps	Intensity	Rest	Notes
Optional: Pogo Jump	3x10	Max Intent	5-10 Secs	Jump as high as you can as fast as you can
Optional: MB CM Chest Throw	4x1	Max Intent	5-10 Secs	Use a 3-5kg MB
BB Back Squat	4x8	RPE 7 65-70%	2-3 Mins	Increase the lift speed during the concentric (upward) phase
DB/BB Lunge	4x8 ES	RPE 7	1-2 Mins	Increase the lift speed during the concentric (upward) phase
BB Bench Press	4x8	RPE 7 65-70%	2-3 Mins	Increase the lift speed during the concentric (upward) phase
Incline DB Press	4x8	RPE 7	1-2 Mins	Increase the lift speed during the concentric (upward) phase
Standing DB/BB Press	4x8	RPE 7	1-2 Mins	Increase the lift speed during the concentric (upward) phase
Single-Leg Calf Raise	3xMax ES	RPE 10	5-10 Secs	Perform with a heel drop
		RPE 7	10-30 Secs	Optional Core: Your choice from page-40

Conditioning Session 1 (CS1):

Activity	Description: Tempo
Run, Row, etc	5km – RPE 7

Program Log 13: Date: ____ / ____ / ____ Day: _____ Time: _____

Exercise	Set 1 WEIGHT		Set 2 WEIGHT		Set 3 WEIGHT		Set 4 WEIGHT		Set 5 WEIGHT	
	REP	RPE	REP	RPE	REP	RPE	REP	RPE	REP	RPE

Conditioning / Notes	Readiness	Bad	Ok	Good
	Sleep:			
	Energy:			
	Mood:			
	Soreness:			

Session RPE: _____

Program Card 14

Phase 3: Intensification – Week-1 (week-7 of the program)

Strength Session 2 (SS2):

Aim to be on your working sets on the primary lift within 3-4 warm-up sets. On Assistance lifts, you can perform 1-2 warm-up sets to groove the movements (if needed).

Exercise	Sets/Reps	Intensity	Rest	Notes
Optional: Bound	3x3 ES	Max Intent	5-10 Secs	Bound from one leg to the other
Optional: MB CM Rotational Throw	3x1 ES	Max Intent	5-10 Secs	Use a 3-5kg MB
BB Deadlift	4x8	RPE 7 65-70%	2-3 Mins	Increase the lift speed during the concentric (upward) phase
DB/BB Lateral Lunge	4x4 ES	RPE 7	1-2 Mins	Increase the lift speed during the concentric (upward) phase
DB/BB Bent-Over Row	4x8	RPE 7	1-2 Mins	Increase the lift speed during the concentric (upward) phase
DB/BB Upright Row	4x8	RPE 7	1-2 Mins	Increase the lift speed during the concentric (upward) phase
DB Single-Arm Row	4x8	RPE 7	1-2 Mins	Increase the lift speed during the concentric (upward) phase
DB/BB Biceps Curl + Triceps Extension	4x8+8	RPE 7	1-2 Mins	Take 5-10 seconds rest between the two exercises – 1-2 deep breaths
		RPE 7	10-30 Secs	Optional Core: Your choice from page-40

Conditioning Session 2 (CS2):

Activity	Description: Intervals	Rest
Run, Row, etc	1x100m – RPE 8	2-3 Mins
	2x200 – RPE 7	3 Mins
	3x400m – RPE 6	3 Min
	1x800m	N/A
Total Distance	2500m	N/A

Program Log 14:   Date: ____ / ____ / ____   Day: _____   Time: _____

Exercise	Set 1 WEIGHT		Set 2 WEIGHT		Set 3 WEIGHT		Set 4 WEIGHT		Set 5 WEIGHT	
	REP	RPE	REP	RPE	REP	RPE	REP	RPE	REP	RPE

Conditioning / Notes	Readiness	Bad	Ok	Good
	Sleep:			
	Energy:			
	Mood:			
	Soreness:			

Session RPE: _____

Program Card 15

Phase 3: Intensification – Week-2 (week-8 of the program)

Strength Session 1 (SS1):

Aim to be on your working sets on the primary lift within 3-4 warm-up sets. On Assistance lifts, you can perform 1-2 warm-up sets to groove the movements (if needed).

Exercise	Sets/Reps	Intensity	Rest	Notes
Optional: Pogo Jump	3x10	Max Intent	5-10 Secs	Jump as high as you can as fast as you can
Optional: MB CM Chest Throw	4x1	Max Intent	5-10 Secs	Use a 3-5kg MB
BB Back Squat	5x5	RPE 8 75-80%	2-3 Mins	Increase the lift speed during the concentric (upward) phase
DB/BB Lunge	4x8 ES	RPE 7	1-2 Mins	Increase the lift speed during the concentric (upward) phase
BB Bench Press	5x5	RPE 8 75-80%	2-3 Mins	Increase the lift speed during the concentric (upward) phase
Incline DB Press	4x8	RPE 7	1-2 Mins	Increase the lift speed during the concentric (upward) phase
Standing DB/BB Press	4x8	RPE 7	1-2 Mins	Increase the lift speed during the concentric (upward) phase
Single-Leg Calf Raise	3xMax ES	RPE 10	5-10 Secs	Perform with a heel drop
		RPE 7	10-30 Secs	Optional Core: Your choice from page-40

Conditioning Session 1 (CS1):

Activity	Description: Tempo
Run, Row, etc	4km – RPE 7-8

Program Log 15: Date: ___ / ___ / ___ Day: _____ Time: _____

Exercise	Set 1		Set 2		Set 3		Set 4		Set 5	
	WEIGHT		*WEIGHT*		*WEIGHT*		*WEIGHT*		*WEIGHT*	
	REP	*RPE*	*REP*	*RPE*	*REP*	*RPE*	*REP*	*RPE*	*REP*	*RPE*

Conditioning / Notes	Readiness	Bad	Ok	Good
	Sleep:			
	Energy:			
	Mood:			
	Soreness:			

Session RPE: _____

Program Card 16

Phase 3: Intensification – Week-2 (week-8 of the program)

Strength Session 2 (SS2):

Aim to be on your working sets on the primary lift within 3-4 warm-up sets. On Assistance lifts, you can perform 1-2 warm-up sets to groove the movements (if needed).

Exercise	Sets/Reps	Intensity	Rest	Notes
Optional: Bound	3x3 ES	Max Intent	5-10 Secs	Bound from one leg to the other
Optional: MB CM Rotational Throw	3x1 ES	Max Intent	5-10 Secs	Use a 3-5kg MB
BB Deadlift	5x5	RPE 8 75-80%	2-3 Mins	Increase the lift speed during the concentric (upward) phase
DB/BB Lateral Lunge	4x4 ES	RPE 7	1-2 Mins	Increase the lift speed during the concentric (upward) phase
DB/BB Bent-Over Row	4x8	RPE 7	1-2 Mins	Increase the lift speed during the concentric (upward) phase
DB/BB Upright Row	4x8	RPE 7	1-2 Mins	Increase the lift speed during the concentric (upward) phase
DB Single-Arm Row	4x8	RPE 7	1-2 Mins	Increase the lift speed during the concentric (upward) phase
DB/BB Biceps Curl + Triceps Extension	4x8+8	RPE 7	1-2 Mins	Take 5-10 seconds rest between the two exercises – 1-2 deep breaths
		RPE 7	10-30 Secs	Optional Core: Your choice from page-40

Conditioning Session 2 (CS2):

Activity	Description: Intervals	Rest
Run, Row, etc	2x100m – RPE 9	2-3 Mins
	2x200 – RPE 8	3 Mins
	3x400m – RPE 7	2 Min
Total Distance	1800m	N/A

Program Log 16: Date: ___ / ___ / ___ Day: _____ Time: _____

Exercise	Set 1 WEIGHT		Set 2 WEIGHT		Set 3 WEIGHT		Set 4 WEIGHT		Set 5 WEIGHT	
	REP	RPE	REP	RPE	REP	RPE	REP	RPE	REP	RPE

Conditioning / Notes	Readiness	Bad	Ok	Good
	Sleep:			
	Energy:			
	Mood:			
	Soreness:			

Session RPE: _____

Program Card 17

Phase 3: Intensification – Week-3 (week-9 of the program)

Strength Session 1 (SS1):

Aim to be on your working sets on the primary lift within 3-4 warm-up sets. On Assistance lifts, you can perform 1-2 warm-up sets to groove the movements (if needed).

Exercise	Sets/Reps	Intensity	Rest	Notes
Optional: Pogo Jump	3x10	Max Intent	5-10 Secs	Jump as high as you can as fast as you can
Optional: MB CM Chest Throw	4x1	Max Intent	5-10 Secs	Use a 3-5kg MB
BB Back Squat	4x3	RPE 8-9 85%	2-3 Mins	Increase the lift speed during the concentric (upward) phase
DB/BB Lunge	4x8 ES	RPE 8	1-2 Mins	Increase the lift speed during the concentric (upward) phase
BB Bench Press	4x3	RPE 8-9 85%	2-3 Mins	Increase the lift speed during the concentric (upward) phase
Incline DB Press	4x8	RPE 8	1-2 Mins	Increase the lift speed during the concentric (upward) phase
Standing DB/BB Press	4x8	RPE 8	1-2 Mins	Increase the lift speed during the concentric (upward) phase
Single-Leg Calf Raise	3xMax ES	RPE 10	5-10 Secs	Perform with a heel drop
		RPE 7	10-30 Secs	Optional Core: Your choice from page-40

Conditioning Session 1 (CS1):

Activity	Description: Tempo
Run, Row, etc	3km – RPE 8-9

Program Log 17:   Date: ____ / ____ / ____   Day: _____   Time: _____

Exercise	Set 1 WEIGHT		Set 2 WEIGHT		Set 3 WEIGHT		Set 4 WEIGHT		Set 5 WEIGHT	
	REP	RPE	REP	RPE	REP	RPE	REP	RPE	REP	RPE

Conditioning / Notes	Readiness	Bad	Ok	Good
	Sleep:			
	Energy:			
	Mood:			
	Soreness:			

Session RPE: _____

Program Card 18

Phase 3: Intensification – Week-3 (week-9 of the program)

Strength Session 2 (SS2):

Aim to be on your working sets on the primary lift within 3-4 warm-up sets. On Assistance lifts, you can perform 1-2 warm-up sets to groove the movements (if needed).

Exercise	Sets/Reps	Intensity	Rest	Notes
Optional: Bound	3x3 ES	Max Intent	5-10 Secs	Bound from one leg to the other
Optional: MB CM Rotational Throw	3x1 ES	Max Intent	5-10 Secs	Use a 3-5kg MB
BB Deadlift	4x3	RPE 9 85%	2-3 Mins	Increase the lift speed during the concentric (upward) phase
DB/BB Lateral Lunge	4x4 ES	RPE 8	1-2 Mins	Increase the lift speed during the concentric (upward) phase
DB/BB Bent-Over Row	4x8	RPE 8	1-2 Mins	Increase the lift speed during the concentric (upward) phase
DB/BB Upright Row	4x8	RPE 8	1-2 Mins	Increase the lift speed during the concentric (upward) phase
DB Single-Arm Row	4x8	RPE 8	1-2 Mins	Increase the lift speed during the concentric (upward) phase
DB/BB Biceps Curl + Triceps Extension	4x8+8	RPE 8	1-2 Mins	Take 5-10 seconds rest between the two exercises – 1-2 deep breaths
		RPE 7	10-30 Secs	Optional Core: Your choice from page-40

Conditioning Session 2 (CS2):

Activity	Description: Intervals	Rest
Run, Row, etc	2x100m – RPE 9	2-3 Mins
	2x200 – RPE 8	3 Mins
	3x400m – RPE 7	2 Min
Total Distance	1800m	N/A

Program Log 18: Date: ___ / ___ / ___ Day: _____ Time: _____

Exercise	Set 1		Set 2		Set 3		Set 4		Set 5	
	WEIGHT		*WEIGHT*		*WEIGHT*		*WEIGHT*		*WEIGHT*	
	REP	RPE	REP	RPE	REP	RPE	REP	RPE	REP	RPE

Conditioning / Notes	Readiness	Bad	Ok	Good
	Sleep:			
	Energy:			
	Mood:			
	Soreness:			

Session RPE: _____

Program Card 19

Phase 4: Realization – Week-1 (week-10 of the program)

Strength Session 1 (SS1):

Aim to be on your working sets on the primary lift within 3-4 warm-up sets. On Assistance lifts, you can perform 1-2 warm-up sets to groove the movements (if needed).

Exercise	Sets/Reps	Intensity	Rest	Notes
Optional: Pogo Jump	3x10	Max Intent	5-10 Secs	Jump as high as you can as fast as you can
Optional: MB Single-Arm Chest Throw	3x1 ES	Max Intent	5-10 Secs	Use a 3-5kg MB – no countermovement
BB Back Squat + VCMJ	3x2+2	RPE 9 85-90%	2-3 Mins	Take 5-10 seconds between the lift and jump (1-2 deep breaths)
DB/BB Lunge	4x6 ES	RPE 8-9	1-2 Mins	Increase the lift speed during the concentric (upward) phase
BB Bench Press + MB Chest Throw	3x2+2	RPE 9 85-90%	2-3 Mins	No countermovement on chest throw
Incline DB Press	4x6	RPE 8-9	1-2 Mins	Increase the lift speed during the concentric (upward) phase
Standing DB/BB Press	4x6	RPE 8-9	1-2 Mins	Increase the lift speed during the concentric (upward) phase
Single-Leg Calf Raise	3xMax ES	RPE 10	5-10 Secs	Perform with a heel drop
		RPE 7	10-30 Secs	Optional Core: Your choice from page-40

Conditioning Session 1 (CS1):

Activity	Description: Tempo
Run, Row, etc	2km – RPE 9

Program Log 19: Date: ____ / ____ / ____ Day: _____ Time: _____

Exercise	Set 1		Set 2		Set 3		Set 4		Set 5	
	WEIGHT		*WEIGHT*		*WEIGHT*		*WEIGHT*		*WEIGHT*	
	REP	RPE	REP	RPE	REP	RPE	REP	RPE	REP	RPE

Conditioning / Notes	Readiness	Bad	Ok	Good
	Sleep:			
	Energy:			
	Mood:			
	Soreness:			

Session RPE: _____

Program Card 20

Phase 4: Realization – Week-1 (week-10 of the program)

Strength Session 2 (SS2):

Aim to be on your working sets on the primary lift within 3-4 warm-up sets. On Assistance lifts, you can perform 1-2 warm-up sets to groove the movements (if needed).

Exercise	Sets/Reps	Intensity	Rest	Notes
Optional: Bound	3x2 ES	Max Intent	5-10 Secs	Bound from one leg to the other
Optional: MB Rotational Throw	3x1 ES	Max Intent	5-10 Secs	Use a 3-5kg MB – no countermovement
BB Deadlift + HCMJ	3x2+2	RPE 9 85-90%	2-3 Mins	Take 5-10 seconds between the lift and jump (1-2 deep breaths)
DB/BB Lateral Lunge	4x3 ES	RPE 8	1-2 Mins	Increase the lift speed during the concentric (upward) phase
DB/BB Bent-Over Row	4x6	RPE 8	1-2 Mins	Increase the lift speed during the concentric (upward) phase
DB/BB Upright Row	4x6	RPE 8	1-2 Mins	Increase the lift speed during the concentric (upward) phase
DB Single-Arm Row	4x6	RPE 8	1-2 Mins	Increase the lift speed during the concentric (upward) phase
DB/BB Biceps Curl + Triceps Extension	4x6+6	RPE 8	1-2 Mins	Take 5-10 seconds rest between the two exercises – 1-2 deep breaths
		RPE 7	10-30 Secs	Optional Core: Your choice from page-40

Conditioning Session 2 (CS2):

Activity	Description: Intervals	Rest
Run, Row, etc	4x100m – 1st RPE 8 / 2nd RPE 9 / 3rd + 4th RPE 10	2-3 Mins
	2x200 – RPE 10	2-3 Mins
Total Distance	800m	N/A

Program Log 20: Date: ____ / ____ / ____ Day: _____ Time: _____

Exercise	Set 1 WEIGHT		Set 2 WEIGHT		Set 3 WEIGHT		Set 4 WEIGHT		Set 5 WEIGHT	
	REP	*RPE*	*REP*	*RPE*	*REP*	*RPE*	*REP*	*RPE*	*REP*	*RPE*

Conditioning / Notes	Readiness	Bad	Ok	Good
	Sleep:			
	Energy:			
	Mood:			
	Soreness:			

Session RPE: _____

Program Card 21

Phase 4: Realization – Week-2 (week-11 of the program)

Strength Session 1 (SS1):

Aim to be on your working sets on the primary lift within 3-4 warm-up sets. On Assistance lifts, you can perform 1-2 warm-up sets to groove the movements (if needed).

Exercise	Sets/Reps	Intensity	Rest	Notes
Optional: Ankle Jump	3x10	Max Intent	5-10 Secs	Jump as high as you can as fast as you can
Optional: MB Single-Arm Chest Throw	3x1 ES	Max Intent	5-10 Secs	Use a 3-5kg MB – no countermovement
BB Back Squat + VCMJ	4x1+2	RPE 9-10 90-95%	2-3 Mins	Take 5-10 seconds between the lift and jump (1-2 deep breaths)
DB/BB Lunge	3x6 ES	RPE 9	1-2 Mins	Increase the lift speed during the concentric (upward) phase
BB Bench Press + MB Chest Throw	4x1+2	RPE 9-10 90-95%	2-3 Mins	No countermovement on chest throw
Incline DB Press	3x6	RPE 9	1-2 Mins	Increase the lift speed during the concentric (upward) phase
Standing DB/BB Press	3x6	RPE 9	1-2 Mins	Increase the lift speed during the concentric (upward) phase
Single-Leg Calf Raise	3xMax ES	RPE 10	5-10 Secs	Perform with a heel drop
		RPE 7	10-30 Secs	Optional Core: Your choice from page-40

Conditioning Session 1 (CS1):

Activity	Description: Tempo
Run, Row, etc	2km – RPE 10

Program Log 21: Date: ____ / ____ / ____ Day: _____ Time: _____

Exercise	Set 1 WEIGHT		Set 2 WEIGHT		Set 3 WEIGHT		Set 4 WEIGHT		Set 5 WEIGHT	
	REP	RPE	REP	RPE	REP	RPE	REP	RPE	REP	RPE

Conditioning / Notes	Readiness	Bad	Ok	Good
	Sleep:			
	Energy:			
	Mood:			
	Soreness:			

Session RPE: _____

Program Card 22

Phase 4: Realization – Week-2 (week-11 of the program)

Strength Session 2 (SS2):

Aim to be on your working sets on the primary lift within 3-4 warm-up sets. On Assistance lifts, you can perform 1-2 warm-up sets to groove the movements (if needed).

Exercise	Sets/Reps	Intensity	Rest	Notes
Optional: Bound	3x2 ES	Max Intent	5-10 Secs	Bound from one leg to the other
Optional: MB Rotational Throw	3x1 ES	Max Intent	5-10 Secs	Use a 3-5kg MB – no countermovement
BB Deadlift + HCMJ	4x1+2	RPE 9-10 90-95%	2-3 Mins	Take 5-10 seconds between the lift and jump (1-2 deep breaths)
DB/BB Lateral Lunge	3x3 ES	RPE 9	1-2 Mins	Increase the lift speed during the concentric (upward) phase
DB/BB Bent-Over Row	3x6	RPE 9	1-2 Mins	Increase the lift speed during the concentric (upward) phase
DB/BB Upright Row	3x6	RPE 9	1-2 Mins	Increase the lift speed during the concentric (upward) phase
DB Single-Arm Row	3x6	RPE 9	1-2 Mins	Increase the lift speed during the concentric (upward) phase
DB/BB Biceps Curl + Triceps Extension	4x6+6	RPE 9	1-2 Mins	Take 5-10 seconds rest between the two exercises – 1-2 deep breaths
		RPE 7	10-30 Secs	Optional Core: Your choice from page-40

Conditioning Session 2 (CS2):

Activity	Description: Intervals	Rest
Run, Row, etc	4x100m – 1st RPE 9 / 2nd + 3rd + 4th RPE 10	2-3 Mins
	1x200 – RPE 10	2-3 Mins
Total Distance	600m	N/A

Program Log 22: Date: ___ / ___ / ___ Day: _____ Time: _____

Exercise	Set 1 WEIGHT		Set 2 WEIGHT		Set 3 WEIGHT		Set 4 WEIGHT		Set 5 WEIGHT	
	REP	RPE	REP	RPE	REP	RPE	REP	RPE	REP	RPE

Conditioning / Notes	Readiness	Bad	Ok	Good
	Sleep:			
	Energy:			
	Mood:			
	Soreness:			

Session RPE: _____

Program Card 23

Phase 4: Realization – Week-3 (week-12 of the program)

Strength Session 1 (SS1):

Aim to be on your working sets on the primary lift within 3-4 warm-up sets. On Assistance lifts, you can perform 1-2 warm-up sets to groove the movements (if needed).

Exercise	Sets/Reps	Intensity	Rest	Notes
Optional: Ankle Jump	3x10	Max Intent	5-10 Secs	Jump as high as you can as fast as you can
Optional: MB Single-Arm Chest Throw	3x1 ES	Max Intent	5-10 Secs	Use a 3-5kg MB – no countermovement
BB Back Squat + VCMJ	3x1+1	RPE 9-10 90-95%	2-3 Mins	Take 5-10 seconds between the lift and jump (1-2 deep breaths)
DB/BB Lunge	3x6 ES	RPE 9	1-2 Mins	Increase the lift speed during the concentric (upward) phase
BB Bench Press + MB Chest Throw	3x1+1	RPE 9-10 90-95%	2-3 Mins	No countermovement on chest throw
Incline DB Press	3x6	RPE 9	1-2 Mins	Increase the lift speed during the concentric (upward) phase
Standing DB/BB Press	3x6	RPE 9	1-2 Mins	Increase the lift speed during the concentric (upward) phase
Single-Leg Calf Raise	3xMax ES	RPE 10	5-10 Secs	Perform with a heel drop
		RPE 7	10-30 Secs	Optional Core: Your choice from page-40

Conditioning Session 1 (CS1):

Activity	Description: Tempo
Run, Row, etc	1km – RPE 10

Program Log 23: Date: ____ / ____ / ____ Day: _____ Time: _____

Exercise	Set 1		Set 2		Set 3		Set 4		Set 5	
	WEIGHT		*WEIGHT*		*WEIGHT*		*WEIGHT*		*WEIGHT*	
	REP	RPE	REP	RPE	REP	RPE	REP	RPE	REP	RPE

Conditioning / Notes	Readiness	Bad	Ok	Good
	Sleep:			
	Energy:			
	Mood:			
	Soreness:			

Session RPE: _____

Program Card 24

Phase 4: Realization – Week-3 (week-12 of the program)

Strength Session 2 (SS2):

Aim to be on your working sets on the primary lift within 3-4 warm-up sets. On Assistance lifts, you can perform 1-2 warm-up sets to groove the movements (if needed).

Exercise	Sets/Reps	Intensity	Rest	Notes
Optional: Bound	3x2 ES	Max Intent	5-10 Secs	Bound from one leg to the other
Optional: MB Rotational Throw	3x1 ES	Max Intent	5-10 Secs	Use a 3-5kg MB – no countermovement
BB Deadlift + HCMJ	3x1+1	RPE 9-10 90-95%	2-3 Mins	Take 5-10 seconds between the lift and jump (1-2 deep breaths)
DB/BB Lateral Lunge	3x3 ES	RPE 9	1-2 Mins	Increase the lift speed during the concentric (upward) phase
DB/BB Bent-Over Row	3x6	RPE 9	1-2 Mins	Increase the lift speed during the concentric (upward) phase
DB/BB Upright Row	3x6	RPE 9	1-2 Mins	Increase the lift speed during the concentric (upward) phase
DB Single-Arm Row	3x6	RPE 9	1-2 Mins	Increase the lift speed during the concentric (upward) phase
DB/BB Biceps Curl + Triceps Extension	4x6+6	RPE 9	1-2 Mins	Take 5-10 seconds rest between the two exercises – 1-2 deep breaths
		RPE 7	10-30 Secs	Optional Core: Your choice from page-40

Conditioning Session 2 (CS2):

Activity	Description: Intervals	Rest
Run, Row, etc	5x100m – 1st RPE 9 / 2nd + 3rd + 4th + 5th RPE 10	2-3 Mins
Total Distance	500m	N/A

Program Log 24: Date: ____ / ____ / ____ Day: _____ Time: _____

Exercise	Set 1 WEIGHT		Set 2 WEIGHT		Set 3 WEIGHT		Set 4 WEIGHT		Set 5 WEIGHT	
	REP	RPE	REP	RPE	REP	RPE	REP	RPE	REP	RPE

Conditioning / Notes	Readiness	Bad	Ok	Good
	Sleep:			
	Energy:			
	Mood:			
	Soreness:			

Session RPE: _____

End of Program Tests

Now that you have completed the 12-week cycle, it is time to test.

If this is the first time you have worked through the program, then this is the first time you will be going through the full testing battery (a testing battery is a group of fitness tests).

There are several ways in which you can complete the tests:

- Perform all the tests in one day (can be split to morning and afternoon)
- Split the tests up over several days – this is optimal

If performing all the tests in one day, follow this protocol:

- **1st Test:** 100m Sprint
- 5-Minutes Rest
- **2nd Test:** Back Squat 1RM
- 5-Minutes Rest
- **3rd Test:** Bench Press 1RM
- 5-Minutes Rest
- **4th Test:** Deadlift 1RM
- 5 Minutes Rest
- **5th Test:** 1-Minute Push-Ups
- 5 Minutes Rest
- **6th Test:** 1-Minute Sit-Ups
- 5-10 Minutes Rest
- **7th Test:** 2km Run or Row
- 5-10 Minutes Rest
- **8th Test:** Max Wall Sit

Note: If performing Pull-Ups or Chin-Ups as a test, perform them prior to the Push-Up test.

If performing the tests on separate days, here are some optimal splits:

Note: Take 5-10 Minutes rests between tests.

Example 1:

Day 1: 100m Sprint + 2km Run or Row
Day 2: Back Squat + Bench Press + Deadlift
Day 3: Push-Ups + Sit-Ups + Wall-Sit

Example 2:

Day 1: 100m Sprint + 2km Run or Row
Day 2: Bench Press
Day 3: Back Squat
Day 4: Deadlift
Day 5: Push-Ups + Sit-Ups + Wall-Sit

Of course, you can vary these splits however suits you best. The main consideration to make is fatigue sensitivity, i.e., You don't want a prior test to have too much of a negative impact on the next test. For example, a Max Wall Sit prior to a 100m sprint or 2km Run is NOT ideal. Whereas a 100m Sprint is not a bad test to carry out prior to a 2km Run as it will potentiate (prime) your body/muscles for the run.

You can carry out basic training during the test week (select assistance exercises from the prior weeks) but be sure to keep the volume and intensity moderate to limit fatigue.

Following the test week, you can jump straight back into the Familiarization phase, which will act as a great deload prior to working through the full 12-weeks to your next test week – use either the novice or intermediate exercises during the 1st phase.

Record all your Test Scores on Page-23

Final Thoughts

Firstly, thanks for downloading a copy of my Youth Strength and Conditioning Program.

If you are an adolescent, then take note of these next 2 paragraphs – if you are a parent or guardian, also take note:

Adolescents are at a time in their life when they can make HUGE improvements in their physical performance. There will never be a stage in their life where they are so adaptable again, so please capitalize on it – all of us 20, 30, 40, 50, 60, 70, 80, 90 and 100-year-olds wish we did!

Take this program, consume the information and work incredibly hard while ensuring you don't train silly and get silly injuries – be consistent, play the long-game and I promise you will look back and be happy you gave yourself the best foundation.

I would love to hear your thoughts on this program (both things you found positive and negative), so please drop me an email at jay@scc.coach and I will answer all emails personally.

Following this page, I have included examples of some of my most popular content – the QR code on the final pages directs you to my LinkTree with over 600-pages of FREE content (you can also check out my books and online courses).

Thanks Again,

Coach Curtis

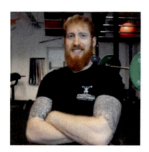

Helpful FREE Content!

Link and QR Code on the last page.

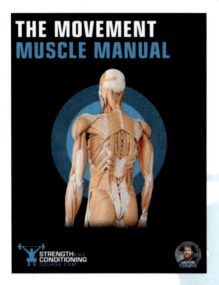

This unique muscle manual categorizes muscles by their movements, giving you a much better understanding of how muscles assist and oppose each other to perform movements.

You also get a FREE second version of the muscle manual, which lists muscle origins, insertions, nerve innervations, etc.

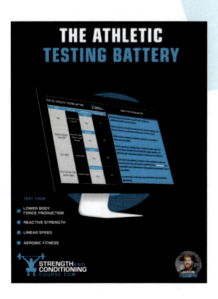

This excel tool tests your lower body force production (vertical countermovement jump), reactive strength (drop jump), linear speed (30m sprint), and aerobic fitness (maximum aerobic speed test).

The tool then creates 4-week targets and generates exercise recommendations.

Helpful FREE Content!

Link and QR Code on the last page.

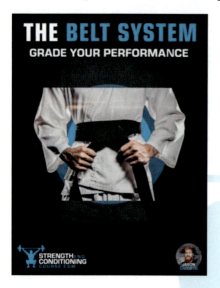

The Belt System was designed as a FUN way for clients and athletes to set targets. However, we were amazed at how popular it became - the increases in motivation have been huge!

There are 5 disciplines, 8 tests per discipline, and 8 coloured belts up for grabs!

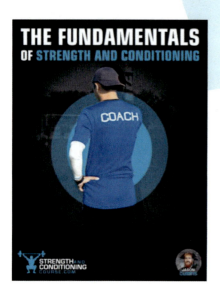

This download takes a look at what it takes to become a strength and conditioning coach and our unique BIG 8 model.

Programming & Periodization / Warming Up / Strength Training / Ballistic Training / Olympic Weightlifting / Plyometrics / Speed & Agility / Metabolic Conditioning.

Online Courses

Link and QR Code on the last page.

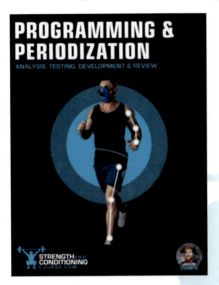

This course details each fundamental step to creating the optimal plan:

The Needs Analysis of both the Sport and Athlete.
Testing of the Athlete.
Analysis of the Results.
Development of the Periodized Plan.
Programming of Sessions.
Evaluations and Modifications.

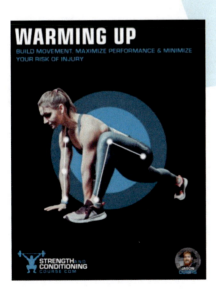

In this course, we delve deeper into how we can optimize the warm-up protocol to minimize our risk of injury and maximize our performance in the subsequent session. We also look at how we create a warm-up that acts as an important part of the session where various physical attributes can be developed long-term.

Online Courses

Link and QR Code on the last page.

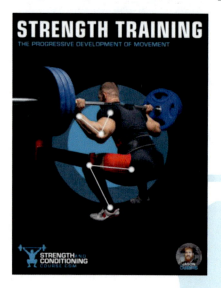

The development of strength is the foundation of physical performance because, before all else, you need the strength in your structures to support the fundamental movements that you carry out each day.

This HUGE course consists of 240+ narrated slides and 4+ hours of video tutorials for over 100 exercises.

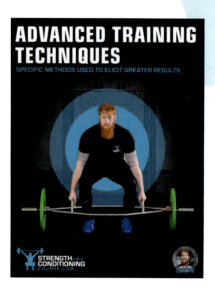

If you want to learn how to smash plateaus and take your training to the next level, this short course is perfect for you.

This course includes over 50 advanced training techniques, many with numerous variations.

A must for those that want greater results!

Books

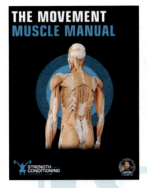 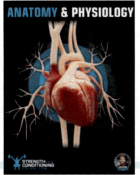 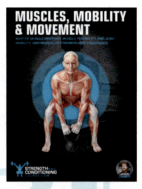

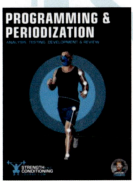 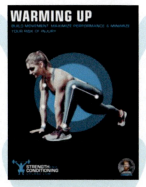 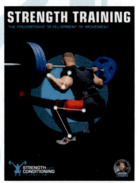

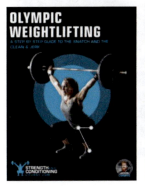 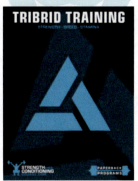 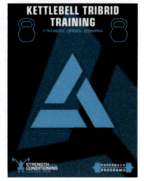

Check out all our content by using the link below or scanning the QR code:

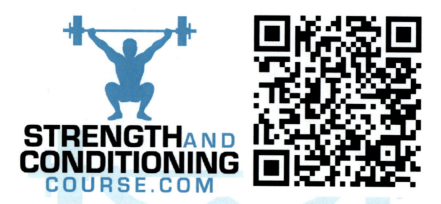

https://courses.strengthandconditioningcourse.com

Purchase any of my other books here:

https://jasoncurtis.org

Scan the QR Code/use the link below to get access to all of my FREE content:

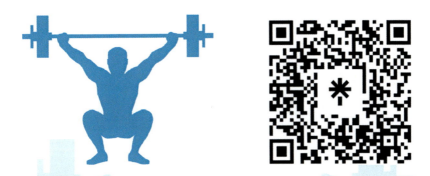

https://linktr.ee/sccacademy

Be social and follow us on our Instagram:

https://instagram.com/strengthandconditioningcourse

Manufactured by Amazon.ca
Bolton, ON

38628978R00062